theclinics.com

DENTAL CLINICS OF NORTH AMERICA

Dentistry's Role in Disaster Response

GUEST EDITOR
Michael D. Colvard, DDS, MTS, MS

October 2007 • Volume 51 • Number 4

SAUNDERS
An Imprint of Elsevier, Inc.
PHILADELPHIA LONDON TORONTO MONTREAL SYDNEY TOKYO

W.B. SAUNDERS COMPANY
A Division of Elsevier Inc.

Elsevier Inc. • 1600 John F. Kennedy Boulevard • Suite 1800 • Philadelphia, Pennsylvania 19103-2899

http://www.dental.theclinics.com

DENTAL CLINICS OF NORTH AMERICA **Volume 51, Number 4**
October 2007 **ISSN 0011-8532**
Editor: John Vassallo; j.vassallo@elsevier.com **ISBN-13: 978-1-4160-5062-9**
ISBN-10: 1-4160-5062-0

Dental Clinics of North America (ISSN 0011-8532) is published quarterly by Elsevier Inc., 360 Park Avenue South, New York, NY 10010-1710. Months of issue are January, April, July, and October. Business and Editorial Offices: 1600 John F. Kennedy Boulevard, Suite 1800, Philadelphia, PA 19103-2899. Customer Service Office: 6277 Sea Harbor Drive, Orlando, FL 32887-4800. Periodicals postage paid at New York, NY and additional mailing offices. Subscription prices are $171.00 per year (US individuals), $281.00 per year (US institutions), $83.00 per year (US students), $204.00 per year (Canadian individuals), $347.00 per year (Canadian institutions), $116.00 per year (Canadian students), $231.00 per year (international individuals), $347.00 per year (international institutions), and $116.00 per year (international students). International air speed delivery is included in all *Clinics* subscription prices. All prices are subject to change without notice. **POSTMASTER:** Send address changes to *Dental Clinics of North America*, Elsevier Periodicals Customer Service, 6277 Sea Harbor Drive, Orlando, FL 32887-4800. Customer Service: 1-800-654-2452 (US). From outside of the US, call 1-407-345-4000.

The Dental Clinics of North America is covered in *Index Medicus, Current Contents/Clinical Medicine, ISI/BIOMED* and *Clinahl.*

Printed in the United States of America.

GUEST EDITOR

MICHAEL D. COLVARD, DDS, MTS, MS, Disaster Emergency Medicine Readiness Training Center; and Department of Oral Medicine and Diagnostic Sciences, College of Dentistry, University of Illinois at Chicago, Chicago, Illinois

CONTRIBUTORS

JOSELI ALVES-DUNKERSON, DDS, MPH, MBA, Olympia, Washington

GEOFFREY A. CORDELL, PhD, Professor Emeritus, Disaster Emergency Medicine Readiness Training Center, College of Dentistry, University of Illinois at Chicago, Chicago, Illinois

PHILLIP L. COULE, MD, FACEP, Associate Professor, Department of Emergency Medicine; and Director, Center of Operational Medicine, Medical College of Georgia, Augusta, Georgia

BENJAMIN GODDER, DMD, Clinical Associate Professor, Department of Cariology and Comprehensive Care, New York University College of Dentistry, New York, New York

DAVID L. GLOTZER, DDS, Clinical Professor, Department of Cariology and Comprehensive Care, New York University College of Dentistry, New York, New York

ALBERT H. GUAY, DMD, Chief Policy Advisor, American Dental Association, Chicago, Illinois

JAMES C. HAGEN, PhD, MBA, MPH, CERC, MEP, Professor; and Director of the Disaster Preparedness and Management Program; and Public and Non-Profit Management Program Graham School of Management, Saint Xavier University, Chicago, Illinois

CHRISTOPHER G. HALLIDAY, DDS, MPH, Chief Dental Officer, US Public Health Service, Indian Health Service, Division of Oral Health, Rockville, Maryland

BERNARD HEILICSER, DO, MS, FACEP, FACOEP, EMS Medical Director for South Cook County; Attending Physician, Ingalls Memorial Hospital, Harvey, Illinois

JACK A. HORNER, BS, President, National Disaster Life Support Foundation, Inc.; Coordinator for Grants, Contracts, and Business Development, Department of Emergency Medicine, Center of Operational Medicine, Medical College of Georgia, Augusta, Georgia

JULIE ANN JANSSEN, RDH, MA, CDHC, Acting Chief, Division of Oral Health, Illinois Department of Public Health, Office of Health Promotion, Springfield, Illinois

LEWIS N. LAMPIRIS, DDS, MPH, Former Chief, Division of Oral Health, Illinois Department of Public Health, Office of Health Promotion, Springfield; Director, Council on Access, Prevention and Interprofessional Relations, American Dental Association, Chicago, Illinois

A. KARL LARSEN, Jr, PhD, Disaster Emergency Medicine Readiness Training Center, College of Dentistry, University of Illinois at Chicago; Toxicology Technical Leader, Illinois State Police, Forensic Sciences Command, Forensic Science Center at Chicago, Chicago, Illinois

MOSES S. LEE, MD, FAAEM, FACEP, Senior Emergency Medicine Attending Physician, John H. Stroger Jr. Hospital of Cook County; Assistant Clinical Professor, Rush Medical University, Chicago, Illinois

FREDERICK G. MORE, DDS, MS, Professor, Department of Epidemiology and Health Promotion; and Department of Pediatric Dentistry, New York University College of Dentistry, New York, New York

NICHOLAS G. MOSCA, DDS, State Dental Director, Division of Health Services, Mississippi State Department of Health; Clinical Professor, Department of Pediatric and Public Health Dentistry, University of Mississippi School of Dentistry, Jackson, Mississippi

MELISSA NAIMAN, MS, EMT-B, Co-Director, Disaster Emergency Medicine Readiness Training Center, College of Dentistry, University of Illinois at Chicago, Chicago, Illinois

BEVERLY PAROTA, RDH, MEd, MBA, CERC, Instructor, Graham School of Management, Saint Xavier University, Chicago; Emergency Response Coordinator, DuPage County Health Department, Wheaton, Illinois

WALTER PSOTER, DDS, PhD, Assistant Professor, Department of Epidemiology and Health Promotion; and Department of Pediatric Dentistry, New York University College of Dentistry, New York, New York; Associate Professor, School of Dentistry, University of Puerto Rico, Puerto Rico

E. DIANNE REKOW, PhD, DDS, Professor and Chair, Department of Basic Science and Craniofacial Biology; and Director of Translational Research, New York University College of Dentistry, New York, New York

CAPT LEE S. SHACKELFORD, DDS, MPA, Executive Assistant to the Assistant Secretary for Health, Office of Public Health and Science, Washington, D.C.

AMY STEWART, MPH, Illinois SNS Director, Division of Disaster Planning & Readiness, Illinois Department of Public Health, Springfield, Illinois

MILA TSAGALIS, RDH, MPH, Dental Health Services Program Manager, DuPage County Health Department, Wheaton, Illinois

PETER R. VALENTIN, MSFS, Disaster Emergency Medicine Readiness Training Center, College of Dentistry, University of Illinois at Chicago, Illinois; Detective, Connecticut State Police, Major Crime Squad, Litchfield, Connecticut

SAMUEL WATSON-ALVÁN, MS, Olympia, Washington

CONTENTS

Foreword xi
CAPT Lee S. Shackelford and Christopher G. Halliday

Preface xv
Michael D. Colvard

The Role Dentists Can Play in Mass Casualty and Disaster Events 767
Albert H. Guay

Dentistry has valuable assets, both in personnel and facilities, to bring to the initial response to a mass casualty event when the local traditional medical system is overwhelmed. This article describes the services dentists can provide to allow physicians to provide the services only they can provide. The education and training of dentists that is required for preparation and the need to develop an integrated emergency response plan are discussed.

Disaster Response in Illinois: The Role for Dentists and Dental Hygienists 779
Julie Ann Janssen and Lewis N. Lampiris

Taking a leadership role, the Illinois Department of Public Health's Division of Oral Health has helped to successfully integrate oral health professionals into the emergency medical response system in Illinois by raising awareness, building needed partnerships, identifying and garnering resources, and facilitating training, policy development, surveillance, and evaluation. Applying the same principals and standards to the integration of oral health and disaster preparedness and response as it does to all facets of dental public health, the division has partnered with the Disaster Emergency Medicine Readiness Training Center at the University of Illinois at Chicago and many other key stakeholders to cement oral health as an integral component to the public health response system in Illinois.

The Importance of a Shared Vision in Emergency Preparedness: Engaging Partners in a Home-Rule State **785**
Samuel Watson-Alván and Joseli Alves-Dunkerson

This article discusses the importance of having a strong vision and culture within the context of emergency preparedness in a home-base state. It proposes a broader vision of public health, one that places public health emergency preparedness and response squarely at the center of the public health mission as a core function. It also lays out work currently underway and the future direction for maximizing the value of response-oriented partnerships at the state and local levels in the Evergreen State. The role of health care professionals and dental providers is specified in more detail. Broadening the public health vision requires recognition of the importance of multisectorial partnerships and their response potential, including the potential roles of all health-related professions and the development of systems to use that potential effectively.

All Hazards Training: Incorporating a Catastrophe Preparedness Mindset into the Dental School Curriculum and Professional Practice **805**
David L. Glotzer, E. Dianne Rekow, Frederick G. More, Benjamin Godder, and Walter Psoter

Catastrophic preparedness should be incorporated into the dental school curriculum. The experience at New York University College of Dentistry is that a combination of catastrophic preparedness elements integrated within existing courses with a short, meaningful capstone course dedicated to all hazards preparedness can be accomplished successfully and meet proposed competencies for training in the dental curriculum. The roles and responsibilities in catastrophic response preparedness and response of dentists are actively being discussed by the dental profession. An element of that discussion has to include the "what" and "how" of education and training for dentists at the predoctoral level and after dental school graduation. The concepts presented in this article should be debated at all levels of the profession.

National Disaster Life Support Programs: A Platform for Multi-Disciplinary Disaster Response **819**
Phillip L. Coule and Jack A. Horner

Proper training must prepare responders to consider various hazards and means by which to mitigate their effects. This article describes one such training program (the National Disaster Life Support program) as a possible means to prepare dental providers to better respond to disasters and describes a simple triage technique that can be used by dental professionals to triage patients.

TOPOFF 2 and the Inclusion of Dental Professionals into Federal Exercise Design and Execution 827
James C. Hagen, Beverly Parota, and Mila Tsagalis

This article examines the dental professional's role in emergency management activities, specifically related to design and execution of such federal exercises as the Top Officials (TOPOFF) series. Experiences from the Chicago TOPOFF 2 exercise are used as an example.

The Role of the Dentist at Crime Scenes 837
Melissa Naiman, A. Karl Larsen, Jr, and Peter R. Valentin

The medical response to a mass casualty further complicates the hectic environment that follows a terrorist event. In addition to providing treatment, medical professionals may discover items or persons of interest to the pending investigation and should be aware of how to handle these situations appropriately. Examples of case law are provided to illustrate how practitioners' actions could help or hinder prosecution. The traditional forensic role of dental professionals is identifying victims through dental records. In this article, the dental professional is considered a member of a disaster response team, and the differences in responsibilities are highlighted.

Pharmaceuticals and the Strategic National Stockpile Program 857
Amy Stewart and Geoffrey A. Cordell

This article discusses current stockpile practices after exploring a history of the use of biologic agents as weapons, the preventive measures that the federal government has used in the past, and the establishment of a Strategic National Stockpile Program in 2003. The article also describes the additional medical supplies from the managed inventory and the federal medical stations. The issues (financial burden, personnel, and materiel selection) for local asset development are also discussed. Critical is the cost to local communities of the development and maintenance of a therapeutic agent stockpile and the need for personnel to staff clinics and medical stations. Finally, the important role of the dental profession for dispensing medication and providing mass immunization in the event of a disaster is described.

Engaging the Dental Workforce in Disaster Mitigation to Improve Recovery and Response 871
Nicholas G. Mosca

Natural disasters may strike quickly and without warning and cause long-term health consequences beyond the immediate loss of lives and property. Dental professionals have a social responsibility to participate in community emergency preparedness planning and response to mitigate prolonged recovery of the dental care infrastructure in the affected areas. Public health and emergency management agencies should plan for access to emergent dental care as part of a multidisciplinary local emergency response to mitigate the impact of devastation on the primary oral health needs of persons in the affected geographic areas. State dental associations should work with government agencies and emergency management groups to increase awareness of the importance for collaborative emergency response health services in the aftermath of natural disasters.

Oral Health Professionals Within State-Sponsored Medical Response Teams: The IMERT Perspective **879**
Moses S. Lee and Bernard Heilicser

In 1999, the State of Illinois recognized the need for a trained and credentialed medical response that can respond to any disaster within the state and will bring health professionals, logistical support, supplies, and equipment to assist local providers when their resources are overwhelmed. The following article reflects on the historical background of the Illinois medical emergency response team, its team development, partnerships, activations, and future directions with the integration of oral health care professionals as a vital resource for emergency response.

Index **895**

FORTHCOMING ISSUES

January 2008

Management of the Oncologic Patient
Sook-Bin Woo, DMD
and Nathaniel S. Treister, DMD, DMSc, *Guest Editors*

April 2008

Dental Public Health
Oscar Arevalo, DDS, MBA
and Amit Chattopadhyay, PhD, MPH, *Guest Editors*

July 2008

Handbook of Dental Practice
Harry Dym, DDS and Orrett Ogle, DDS, *Guest Editors*

RECENT ISSUES

July 2007

Dental Materials
Lyle D. Zardiackas, PhD, FADM,
Tracy M. Dellinger, DDS, MS,
and Mark Livingston, DDS, *Guest Editors*

April 2007

Successful Esthetic and Cosmetic Dentistry for the Modern Dental Practice
John R. Calamia, DMD, Mark S. Wolff, DDS, PhD,
and Richard J. Simonsen, DDS, MS, *Guest Editors*

January 2007

Temporomandibular Disorders and Orofacial Pain
Henry A. Gremillion, DDS, *Guest Editor*

ELSEVIER
SAUNDERS

THE DENTAL CLINICS OF NORTH AMERICA

Dent Clin N Am 51 (2007) xi–xiii

Foreword

The subject of dental forensics has been recognized for decades as an area of emphasis for all interested and properly trained dentists in all hazards response. Additionally, the US Military and other entities within the federal government have recognized a role in the areas of emergency readiness and response for dentists for several years, but these subjects have not been on the forefront of awareness for most—until September 11, 2001.

Since then, professional dental organizations, schools of dentistry, individual authors, and other entities have emphasized dentistry's roles in emergency preparedness and response, bio-response, vaccination/immunization, disease surveillance, and other related activities. The Academy of General Dentistry (AGD) published an AGD Impact issue that highlighted roles played by AGD dentists in the September 11 aftermath [1]. In June 2002, the American Dental Association (ADA) convened a workshop titled, *Dentistry's Response to Bioterrorism*. Dr. Al Guay reported on the meeting in September 2002 [2].

In March 2003, the ADA and US Public Health Service (USPHS) collaborated to present *Dentistry's Role in Responding to Bioterrorism and Other Catastrophic Events*, a meeting that was attended by oral health and dental professionals from the Department of Defense, USPHS, numerous other federal agencies and operating divisions, representatives from organized dentistry, dental academia, and state, local, and other public health entities. At that meeting, United States Surgeon General, Vice Admiral Richard Carmona emphasized, "Dentists have a role in emergency response because they have the patient care skills, medical knowledge and communication skills."

At the same conference, Dr. Michael Alfano, Dean of the New York University College of Dentistry, spoke in support of an immunization and inoculation role for dentists. Illustrating his point with a picture of the needle tip on a dental syringe poised at the mandibular foramen on the bare mandible of a skull, he stated, "If you can hit this..." followed by a slide of a bare triceps injection site, "... you can hit this!"

For a time there seemed to be a groundswell of emergency preparedness awareness courses, casualty treatment and disaster response workshops, and articles presented by a variety of dental professional organizations and journals highlighting potential roles for dentists. An April 2006 article in the Journal of the American Dental Association (JADA) cited, from a variety of journals, 15 separate references that addressed the emergency response

0011-8532/07/$ - see front matter
doi:10.1016/j.cden.2007.06.008

role of dentists or dentistry. Those citations did not include references to dental forensics, which, for decades, has been a discipline within the oral health community and has been a well-accepted role for dentists.

During the summer of 2005, with the devastating hurricanes that struck the Gulf States, another facet in the role of dentists and dentistry in emergency response and event mitigation came to the collective consciousness of oral health professionals: could dentistry have roles that are deeper than forensics, patient counseling, and other public health roles?

In April 2006, JADA published an article written by several contributors that spelled out the process that occurred in Illinois, where an expanded role of "Dental Emergency Responder" has been written into the Illinois State Dental Practice Act [3]. Within the article was a description of a program developed by the American Medical Association through its Center for Public Health Preparedness and Disaster Response: the National Disaster Life Support (NDLS) program. Within the NDLS protocols there are clear roles that can be filled by properly trained dentists.

Having dentists named as potential participants in such a program enhances the credibility that properly trained dentists should have a proper role in disaster response. There are other disaster response protocols that do not currently recognize dentistry by name as potential participants (eg, the National Incident Management System and other command protocols). Issues such as the *Dental Clinics of North America* that highlight the voids in dental representation in disaster response programs may go far in disseminating the concept that the time has arrived for dentists and other properly trained oral health professionals to be full participants in recognized disaster response efforts.

CAPT Lee S. Shackelford, DDS, MPA
Executive Assistant to the Assistant Secretary for Health
Office of Public Health and Science
Hubert H. Humphrey Building
Rm. 701H, 200 Independence Ave. SW
Washington, DC 20201, USA

E-mail address: lee.shackelford@hhs.gov

Christopher G. Halliday, DDS, MPH
Chief Dental Officer
US Public Health Service
Indian Health Service
Division of Oral Health
Suite 300, 801 Thompson Avenue
Rockville, MD 20852, USA

E-mail address: christopher.halliday@ihs.gov

References

[1] Mages M. Are you prepared? Sept. 11 tragedy called on dentists in ways few could have imagined. AGD Impact 2002;30(3):8–10.
[2] Guay A. Dentistry's response to bioterrorism: a report of a consensus workshop. J Am Dent Assoc 2002;133(9):1181–7.
[3] Colvard MD, Lampiris LN, Cordell GA, et al. The dental emergency responder; expanding the scope of dental practice. J Am Dent Assoc 2006;137(4):468–73.

ELSEVIER
SAUNDERS

THE DENTAL CLINICS OF NORTH AMERICA

Dent Clin N Am 51 (2007) xv–xvii

Preface

Dentists and dental hygienists, as individuals and members of professions, have demonstrated records of professional volunteerism and contribution at all levels of the community, state, federal, and political arenas in the United States and the world. The dental profession is one of the most highly regarded and socially active of health care professions. Dentistry enjoys a public status that is recognized as a significant system of health care and a professional autonomy, collaborating with the professions of medicine, nursing, public health, and information sciences. Dentists have the opportunity for specialization, including surgery and public health; each individual dentist actively elects how he/she will practice dentistry. The clinical skill sets and infrastructure that the dental profession can bring to support community needs is singularly impressive.

As the magnitude of man-made and natural disasters increase in scope and destruction, the local availability of first responders and infrastructures available to political decision makers becomes paramount. If the local assets are overwhelmed, the expectations for response within the community change. The role of traditional first responders shifts particularly during a disaster, when assets are exceeded, which possibly causes the role of the oral health professional to shift as well. The nature and extent of this shift requires an examination of the expansion of the definition of first responders and an assessment of the validity of the inclusion of the dental profession as significant contributors within the domain of the first responder community.

For example, in Illinois, while the initial idea to create the "Dental Emergency Responder" as part of the Illinois Dental Practice Act came from the Illinois Department of Public Health Division of Oral Health, a great deal of the legislative legwork was driven by the state dental society. Other states currently are pursuing similar legislative definitions to protect the interests of dental professionals, and these measures will be successful only with the support of individual practitioners on many levels.

Preparedness, in its nature, is multifaceted and requires a great deal of creativity to overcome the limitations imposed in the use of expected or traditional assets. This issue chronicles the view of numerous dental professionals who have demonstrated careers in public health and community responses, especially in the domain of first response to man-made and/or natural disasters. Each author details experiences related to the participation

doi:10.1016/j.cden.2007.07.003

dental.theclinics.com

of oral health professionals across the country in disaster response over the past five years. Readers will observe that the dental profession has been involved in this new first responder paradigm for many years and on many fronts, including policy, education, drills, and team training. The scope of experiences demonstrated here helps to frame the definition of potential roles for oral health care professionals in disaster medicine response. All authors agree that there is a profound role for dentistry in the disaster response paradigm, both in personnel and infrastructure support. Hygienists, dentists, and dental specialists can bring a wide range of skill sets based on personal experience, training, and enthusiasm. The oral health community offers skilled manpower and orthogonal medical supply caches, which provide a high-impact contribution to disaster planning and management activities. However, members of public health, emergency planning, and other stakeholders must be encouraged to include the dental profession in their tactical and strategic planning, and they must be educated about the potential roles oral health professionals see for themselves.

Hurdles remain, because the majority of the disaster medicine and response community naturally does not perceive a contributing role by the dental profession. Therefore, it remains imperative for the oral health community as a whole to continue to be active participants in all aspects of preparedness involving disaster medicine and response education to participation. If the dental profession does not become involved and partner with the disaster medicine and response community, noninvolvement will lead to a complete inability to participate. We must make the case to the disaster medicine and response community that the dental profession can participate and should be perceived to belong within the disaster medicine and response domain. Becoming involved in disaster medicine readily can be seen as an extension of dental practice. As dentists recognize oral manifestations of systemic ailments and offer appropriate intervention and follow-up measures, dentists also can become familiar with the various manifestations of exposure to chemical and biological agents, provide initial intervention, and recommend appropriate advanced care. In order to have this opportunity, however, the entire dental community must remain involved in discussions around policy, planning, and implementation to shape the image of the role of the dentist and dental hygienist within medicine and response.

With the recent passage of the anniversary of September 11, many questions about the past and the future resurfaced, particularly whether or not our nation is prepared, and what preparedness means. Each segment of our society should contribute to the answer and the definition, because an effective response will come only from community-wide acceptance of the actions required to respond. On a personal level, involvement in the health and welfare of the community reconfirms the role of the dentist in overall health care. On an ethical level, dental professionals who provide public health and community care to those in need fulfill one of the primary tenants of medicine. In reading this issue, it is the authors' hope that the dental community will be inspired by the successes, will be better prepared for the difficulties, and will be ready to support the concept of dentistry's role within disaster response.

Michael D. Colvard, DDS, MTS, MS
Disaster Emergency Medicine Readiness Training Center
Department of Oral Medicine and Diagnostic Sciences
College of Dentistry
University of Illinois at Chicago
801 S. Paulina Street, Room 569D
Chicago, IL 60612, USA

E-mail address: colvard@uic.edu

ELSEVIER
SAUNDERS

THE DENTAL CLINICS OF NORTH AMERICA

Dent Clin N Am 51 (2007) 767–778

The Role Dentists Can Play in Mass Casualty and Disaster Events

Albert H. Guay, DMD

American Dental Association, 211 East Chicago Avenue, Chicago, IL 60611-2678, USA

It is evident from recent catastrophic events that the traditional medical care system may be overwhelmed because many medical centers operate close to capacity on a daily basis. Add the generation of mass casualties by a major incident or a significant bioterrorism attack into the equation, and a basic life-saving response by the existing medical care system becomes nearly impossible. Unfortunately, the current world geopolitical environment makes such a scenario entirely possible—some say inevitable. There is a need to marshal all available resources in response to a disaster of great magnitude if losses and disruption of everyday life are to be minimized and recovery facilitated.

Professionals who plan and manage emergency responses must reach out to groups that have assets to contribute to the response effort but are not intrinsically tied to the medical response (eg, hospital personnel). Dentists and dental staff are examples of such groups. For a long time, dentistry has played a well-acknowledged role in participating in the recovery from mass casualty events, such as natural disasters, bombings, and transportation accidents, primarily in the forensic identification of victims when identities cannot be established by conventional means. Some individual dentists also have participated in victim rescue and treatment.

For the most part, the dental profession is a loosely organized network of individual practitioners. There are approximately 175,000 professionally active dentists in the United States, and they are distributed in a manner much like that of the general population [1]. They own, equip, and supply the office facilities in which they provide oral health care. Approximately 85% of dental practices in the United States are solo practices, and 11% are made up of two dentists [2]. The consolidation that has characterized many industries and businesses in the United States, including medicine,

E-mail address: guaya@ada.org

0011-8532/07/$ - see front matter
doi:10.1016/j.cden.2007.06.002 ***dental.theclinics.com***

has not occurred in dentistry. Only a small proportion of dental care is provided in a hospital setting. In contrast to medicine, most dental care is provided to patients by one primary care dentist in one facility. The average dental office is essentially a mini-hospital or an outpatient clinic. It is equipped with radiographic capability, sterilization equipment, central suction, medical gasses and various anesthesia capabilities, suites with surgical lighting, some surgical equipment and supplies, laboratory space, and administrative areas for records and patient reception. Trained and experienced office staff are present to operate in these areas. Dental offices are dispersed throughout the community.

Dentists are exposed to information in many general medical areas during their predoctoral education that can be useful in disaster response situations. They also routinely perform many tasks that emergency responders may be required to do, such as perform minor surgery, dispense drugs, give injections, and administer anesthesia. It should be apparent from this description that dentistry has much to contribute to the response to a major disaster in terms of personnel and facilities when the traditional medical care system in an area is overwhelmed. This article describes how dentists and allied dental staff can help respond to major disasters.

After the seminal events that occurred in the fall 2001, particularly the deliberate attempts to spread weapons-grade *Bacillus anthracis* spores through the US mail system [3], the American Dental Association convened two workshops to determine how dentistry could contribute to the response to mass casualty disasters and how dentistry could become better prepared to respond: (1) a workshop on the role of dentistry in bioterrorism [4], cosponsored by the US Public Health Service, and (2) a workshop on terrorism and mass casualty curriculum development [5], cosponsored by the American Dental Education Association. A wide variety of emergency response experts and stakeholders in dentistry attended these workshops. Consensus was reached at these workshops on both subjects, including plans for implementing the suggestions that were developed. Because responses to these disasters are directed by local emergency response agencies, it was determined that the responsibility for dental participation in the response effort must lie with the local dental societies. They were promised to receive assistance and advice from the American Dental Association in developing and organizing dentistry's response. They also were advised that any plans they develop must be done with the participation of the local emergency response community so that the dental response plan can be fully integrated into the local plan.

It is generally thought that dentistry can be of greatest assistance immediately after the occurrence of a mass disaster before the full force of federal assistance can be mobilized effectively. During recent disasters, this mobilization time varied from a few days to a week. Many victims of disasters cannot wait that long for help. When local medical resources are unable to cope adequately with a huge number of victims, dentists can be recruited to provide certain services that will allow physicians to do things only they can do. Dentists can enhance the surge capacity of the local medical system until additional physicians arrive or the demand for immediate care decreases.

How dentists can help

The prime purpose of recruiting the assistance of dentists in responding to mass casualty incidents is to enable crisis managers to use scarce physician resources in the most effective manner possible by having some services they would ordinarily provide be successfully provided by dentists where possible. Local circumstances (ie, the medical needs and resources of the community after a disaster and the nature of the disaster) determine how dentists can be of assistance. Some assigned duties do not tax the dentist's knowledge or experience (eg, dispensing medications or immunizations), whereas others may require additional training or some supervision (eg, providing basic medical care in quarantine situations). There are several general areas of response activity in which dentists can be helpful [4].

Surveillance

Some mass casualty events are distinct entities easily recognized and of easily defined duration and effect on a population (eg, a severe weather event). Other disasters, particularly bioterrorism attacks and pandemics, often have relatively indistinguishable beginnings and ends and unpredictable effects on a population. Because of the variable incubation periods of infectious agents, the time of exposure can be estimated only after the resultant disease has manifested. It also may take up valuable time to determine that a population-wide problem actually exists. Dentists can be part of an effective surveillance network because they are scattered throughout a community much as the general population is and are visited by patients who are generally medically healthy and have not seen a physician. Observation of intraoral or cutaneous lesions or both when they are present and the notification of public health authorities about these observations may facilitate the early detection of a bioterrorism attack or spread of a pandemic infection. Early detection of an infectious agent in a population may allow for reduction in the number of casualties by prompt initiation of preventive and therapeutic intervention.

Sales of over-the-counter medications are often monitored in the epidemiology community as a potential early warning of community-wide infections. Monitoring of unusual and unexplained "no show" patients in dental offices also may help provide an early warning. A reporting network and a real-time analytic mechanism involving other inputs also must be established for this to be of value in early detection.

Referral of patients

Patients who show early signs or symptoms of infectious diseases, have suspicious cutaneous lesions, or are suspected of having such diseases may be referred to a physician for a definitive diagnosis and appropriate treatment, if necessary. This referral may be important because early treatment or early initiation of prophylaxis can have a significant influence on the outcome of the patient's encounter with the disease. The clinical course of smallpox, for example, can be ameliorated by vaccination even after the patient has been infected.

Diagnosis and monitoring

After an infectious disease that causes mass casualties has been identified, dentists who are able to recognize the signs and symptoms of that disease may be able to identify afflicted patients. Dentists can collect salivary samples, nasal swabs, or other specimens when appropriate for laboratory processing that may yield valuable diagnostic information or indication of the progress of treatment, including the status of the patient's infectiousness.

Triage

In the effective response to any mass casualty event a system must be established to prioritize treatment among casualties, because immediate treatment for all casualties is not possible because of inadequate resources in personnel, facilities, and medical supplies. Dentists are able to assist in this important function with relatively little additional training. This assistance allows physicians to provide definitive care for patients most urgently in need rather than screening casualties. Dental offices could serve as triage centers if needed.

Immunizations

To limit the spread of infectious agents, whether from a natural pandemic, a deliberate bioterrorism attack, or contamination as a result of a local event, rapid immunization of great numbers of individuals may be required in a short amount of time. In major metropolitan areas, where the spread of communicable disease is facilitated, this effort may involve millions of people. Physicians and nurses may be unable to implement such a program in the critical time frame required. Dentists can participate in mass immunization programs with a minimum of additional training and may be the critical factor in the success of urgent programs. Dental offices can be used as immunization sites to minimize the concentration of potentially infected persons.

Medications

In mass casualty situations, particularly after a bioterrorism attack or the unfolding of a pandemic infection, the population may require medication to treat or prevent the manifestation of the infection being faced. Physicians, nurses, and pharmacists may not be able to effectively prescribe or dispense the medications necessary in the critical, appropriate time required. Dentists can be called on to prescribe and dispense the medications required after that determination has been made by the physicians and public health officials managing the disease outbreak. Dentists also can monitor patients for adverse reactions and side effects and refer patients who experience untoward effects from the medications to physicians for treatment, if necessary. Dentists also can be used as sources of information for patients concerning the medications they are using by communicating information on proper use, problems that may occur and their manifestation, and the need for compliance. Dentists can monitor the effectiveness of the treatment regimen.

Infection control

Dentists and dental auxiliaries practice sound infection control procedures in their offices on a daily basis. They are well versed and well practiced in infection control and can bring their expertise to mass casualty situations, particularly situations that involve infectious agents, to limit the spread of infection among individuals and between patients and responders who are rendering assistance. Decontamination of casualties from certain bioterrorism attacks in which contact with patients' clothing or skin surfaces may spread the agent to caregivers may be accomplished by dentists with some additional training. Dentists who are familiar with disaster mortuary activities can be useful in managing the remains of victims whose death is a result of the event, particularly infectious events. These remains most likely will be contaminated and require careful management to prevent further disease spread.

Definitive treatment

In addition to providing services that dentists ordinarily do, they may be able to augment or participate in the treatment provided by medical and surgical personnel. Dentists have training and experience in many areas that may be a part of casualty care in mass casualty events:

- Treating oral, facial, and cranial injuries
- Providing cardiopulmonary resuscitation
- Obtaining medical histories
- Collecting blood and other samples
- Providing or assisting with anesthesia
- Starting intravenous lines

- Suturing and performing appropriate surgery
- Assisting in patient stabilization
- Assisting in shock management

Quarantine

During a pandemic or after a bioterrorism attack with a communicable agent, strict quarantine restrictions may be imposed on the geographic area contaminated and its environs to help prevent or control the spread of the disease to other areas. The duration of the quarantine varies according to the incubation time of the agent and other factors. Before the existence of the area-wide contamination is established, primary care providers may become infected directly or through contact with patients seeking care. During the period of quarantine they may become disabled by the disease or even die. Dentists may not be similarly infected by patients because ill patients do not seek care from dentists and, if sufficiently ill, do not keep scheduled dental appointments, which minimizes intimate contact with infected persons. Dentists may be called on to provide some primary health care for people in the quarantined area.

After the initial response

When federal assistance arrives and the surge in immediate medical care needs subsides to the point that local medical systems are able to accommodate community requirements, the role that dentists can play changes. The original strategy of having dentists substitute where possible for physicians in the acute initial stress situation is replaced by a strategy that has dentists extending the system's reach and capacity beyond that of the traditional medical care system over an extended period of time. In the case of an infectious disease that causes mass casualties, dentists can provide an extensive surveillance network that may be able to identify potential infection spreading in areas beyond the original contaminated area and trigger extensive preventive measures to control the spread. Dentists also may be able to spot the re-emergence of infections in areas previously considered to be under control. Dentistry should participate actively in the emergency, public health, and medical community postevent analyses to determine how the immediate response to mass casualty events can be improved and how dentistry's role can be enhanced.

How dental auxiliaries can help

Confusion, disorganization, and lack of control are major barriers to an effective response to a mass casualty event. Experienced personnel are required to establish and maintain as orderly a process as possible for the immediate response to avoid public panic. Dental office clerical personnel are experienced in administrative functions, managing medical records, organizing patient flow, and maintaining communications between dentists and other health care providers. They can provide valuable assistance in those areas. Dental assistants can retain their role in assisting dentists, even expanding their function under supervision to help dentists in the new roles they may be asked to fill. Dental hygienists can provide new clinical services with additional training, perhaps including administering immunizations in mass disaster immunization programs.

The role of dental societies

Mass casualty events usually occur in defined areas. Because the disaster event usually begins as a local phenomenon, the initial response also is local. Management of the response is the responsibility of a designated local emergency response agency that has developed and tested an emergency response plan designed specifically for the local area. The plan uses a combination of immediately available local assets and resources that become available in varying lengths of time from state and federal agencies.

Dental societies should develop a disaster response plan for dentists to provide community assistance in the event of a mass casualty situation [6]. That plan should be developed with the cooperation of the local emergency response and public health communities and should be integrated fully into local emergency response plans. It may be advisable to have a representative from the local emergency response community serve as a consultant to the dental society as the society plan is developed and appoint a dental society representative to attend local planning meetings. The nature and extent of the plan vary according to local conditions, dental society resources, and the willingness of dentists in the area to participate. Components of the plan are shown in Box 1.

In smaller states, one dentistry-centric disaster response plan may be sufficient and the state dental society can develop it and provide all the services required to maintain the plan. In heavily populated states, several plans may be required, involving component dental societies and the constituent dental society in their development and maintenance. The American Dental Association has developed and distributed to the state dental societies a template that may be used in developing a dental response plan. That template is still available from the American Dental Association to any organization that requests it. Technical advice and consultation are also available from the American Dental Association for local dental societies on any aspect of responding to mass casualty disaster events.

How to prepare the profession

Besides developing a disaster response plan for dentistry's response to mass casualty disasters, the profession itself must be made aware of the

Box 1. Components of a disaster response plan

Purpose: Explanation of why the plan has been developed and to what use it should be put.

Glossary of terms: Because much of the "emergency" terminology may be new to the average dentist, definitions are important for all to have a clear understanding of the information presented.

Situation and assumptions: Clear description of the situations in which the plan is implemented and the assumptions made about the situation that have been made in developing the plan.

Organization and responsibilities: Description of the organizational structure to support development of the plan, its implementation and periodic review, and the resources to be allocated and a delineation of the duties and responsibilities of individuals involved. An emergency response manager should be designated and a reporting hierarchy constituted.

Command, control, and communications: The command and control structure of the dental response plan should be integrated completely into the local disaster management structure. Communications, a critical part of management, should be established and tested periodically.

Volunteer coordination: A survey should be conducted to determine the skill and experience levels of dentists willing to participate in response activities so that an inventory of assets the dental society can bring to emergency situations can be developed.

Liaison with disaster agencies: It is imperative that ongoing liaison with the appropriate local disaster agencies and joint operations centers be established.

Specific assistance activities: Catalog of activities made available to local emergency response organizations.

Training and exercises: Plan development alone does not guarantee an effective response. Periodic training and mock exercises that include responders from many disciplines should be included.

Review and update: The plan should be reviewed and updated regularly.

added responsibilities it may be asked to take on if traditional medical resources of the community are swamped by a surge in demand for care in the wake of a large-scale disaster. Additional education and training for dentists in specific areas of emergency response that build on the basic principles of medical care with which they are familiar can significantly expand the scope of services that dentists can provide effectively during these emergencies. Educational efforts should begin with dental students in during their predoctoral education [5]. The curriculum should be expanded to include more information on the management of large numbers of casualties, especially casualties generated by the intentional or nonintentional spread of infectious agents. Dental students should understand the public health and emergency response communities and the control functions they provide in the event of an emergency. This material can be presented in separate dedicated courses or combined with appropriate existing course work. In either case it is advisable to have a separate course in the last year of dental school that pulls together all of the information taught during the preceding years as a summary.

In addition to the teaching of dental students, the existing profession needs similar education and training [7], which presents more of an educational challenge because of the practice responsibilities of dentists in the community and their ability to abstain from participation. As such, for the near future, most dentists who may be called on to assist in disaster response efforts most likely will not have received formal disaster training. The task of educating dental students falls primarily on dental schools. Educating and training dental practitioners is not as centralized as for dental students and must be accomplished by various means and from various sources, including dental schools, more than likely coordinated through the dental societies. State licensing agencies also may play a role in dental provider education in this area. There are opportunities for dentists who are interested in going beyond basic education and training in responding to mass casualty events through participation in various organizations sponsored by state and federal emergency response agencies.

There has been some discussion about whether the education and training of dentists in bioterrorism and mass casualty response should be mandatory or optional. The American Dental Association would like to see this education mandatory in dental schools. The State of Nevada has required that all candidates for initial licensure or license renewal as dentists or dental hygienists complete 6 hours of education in bioterrorism and mass casualty events. The American Dental Association-United States Public Health Service workshop adopted an education and training preparatory plan that is represented in Fig. 1. It suggests mandatory education and training in the basic capabilities that are required when dentists respond to a mass casualty event. Preparation beyond the basic skills needed or certification credentialing should be voluntary.

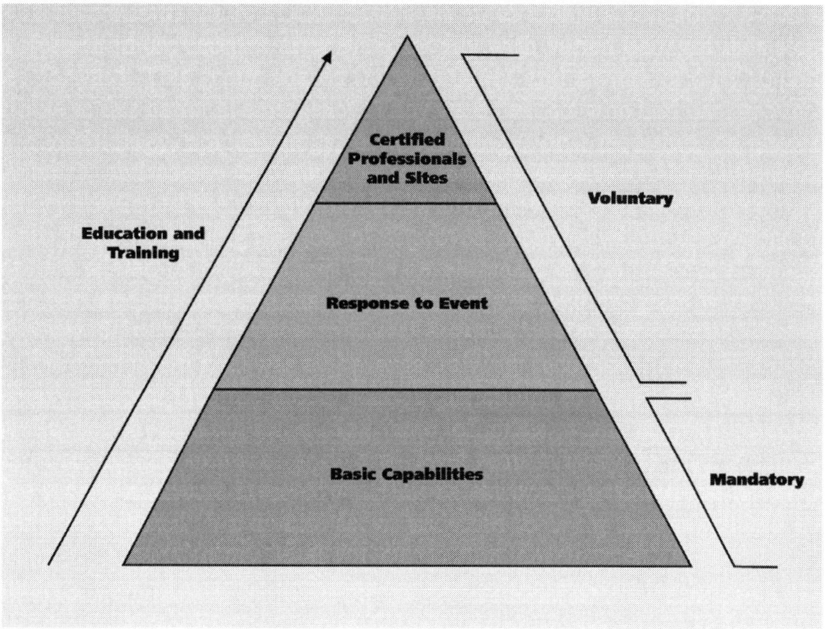

Fig. 1. A schematic representation of dentists' educational preparation for and participation in responding to a bioterrorism attack, as proposed by participants in the American Dental Association's Workshop on the Role of Dentistry in Bioterrorism. (*From* Guay AH. Dentistry's response to bioterrorism: a report of a consensus workshop. JADA 2002;133:1181–7; with permission.)

Legal and licensure issues

Several legal and licensure issues must be addressed and resolved favorably if there is to be any chance of significant participation by dentists in the emergency response to mass casualty events. The major issues are licensure, scope of practice and credentialing, and the legal liability of responders.

Licensure

Mass casualty events, particularly those related to the spread of infectious diseases, do not respect political boundaries. In a declared emergency, dentists should be able to cross state lines to render care without concern for the geographic limitations on their right to practice imposed by state licensure. Some mechanism must be established to eliminate these restrictions or valuable human resources may be wasted at a time when they are needed most. This exemption is usually provided for "medical responders" through a temporary exemption from licensure requirements during a declared emergency. Dentists are not generally considered to be "medical responders." The role of dentists as emergency medical responders should be codified so they can assist in responding to catastrophic events with the usual exemptions.

Scope of practice and credentialing

It should be clear that dentists may be called on to provide services that are beyond the normal scope of dental practice in a mass casualty event. In a declared emergency, the strict scope of dental practice outlined in state dental practice acts must relaxed to enable dentists to provide services that they are able to provide and are in great demand during the duration of the emergency. Credentialing dentists to delineate which services they may provide in an emergency is likely to discourage many dentists from becoming volunteer responders and may waste critically needed medical resources. Credentialing dentists who choose to be a part of an organized response team is appropriate, however, because they most likely would be assigned to provide a higher level of services than the average dentist who volunteers to be of assistance in an emergency. Checking the credentials of a volunteer dentist or any health care volunteer may be close to impossible during the initial surge demand period.

Legal liability

Because dental responders to mass casualty events may be practicing in an area in which they are not licensed and are providing services beyond the legal scope of dental practice and for which they are not credentialed, there must be legal relief from liability for their acts or omissions for responders who act in good faith and as an average dentist faced with the same circumstances would act. Failure to provide relief from liability for dentists who respond to a mass casualty event will have a severe dampening effect on the recruitment of dentist volunteers. It will significantly reduce the number of dentists who obtain predisaster education and training because they would not plan to volunteer to assist.

Summary

Dentistry has valuable assets in personnel and facilities to contribute to the response to a mass casualty event, particularly one that results from the spread of disease through the population. The dental profession and emergency response communities should work together to maximize the effectiveness of dentistry's contribution and prepare the dental community to be effective responders.

References

[1] American Dental Association, Survey Center. Distribution of dentists in the United States by region and state, 2004. Chicago: American Dental Association; 2006.

[2] American Dental Association, Survey Center. 2005 survey of dental practice: characteristics of dentists in private practice and their patients. Chicago: American Dental Association; 2007.
[3] Flores S, Mills SE, Shackelford L. Dentistry and bioterrorism. Dent Clin North Am 2003;47: 733–44.
[4] Guay AH. Dentistry's response to bioterrorism: a report of a consensus workshop. J Am Dent Assoc 2002;133:1181–7.
[5] Chmar JE, Ranney RR, Guay AH, et al. Incorporating bioterrorism training into dental education: report of ADA-ADEA terrorism and mass casualty curriculum development workshop. J Dent Educ 2004;68(11):1196–9.
[6] American Dental Association. Dentistry's response to bioterrorism and other mass disasters. Chicago: American Dental Asociation; 2003.
[7] Colvard MD, Lampiris LN, Cordell GA, et al. The dental emergency responder: expanding the scope of dental practice. J Am Dent Assoc 2006;137:468–73.

ELSEVIER
SAUNDERS

Dent Clin N Am 51 (2007) 779–784

THE DENTAL CLINICS OF NORTH AMERICA

Disaster Response in Illinois: The Role for Dentists and Dental Hygienists

Julie Ann Janssen, RDH, MA, CDHC[a,*], Lewis N. Lampiris, DDS, MPH[b,1]

[a]*Division of Oral Health, Illinois Department of Public Health, Office of Health Promotion, 535 W. Jefferson St., Springfield, IL 62761, USA*

[b]*Council on Access, Prevention and Interprofessional Relations, American Dental Association, Chicago, IL, USA*

The critical nature of emergency response came into sharp focus for the Illinois Department of Public Health's (IDPH) oral health staff on September 11, 2001, when the state's first Oral Health Summit was cut short by news of the terrorist attack in New York City. Instead of discussing strategies to implement the oral health plan they were ratifying, summit participants dispersed. Many, including several state leaders, were summoned to quickly respond to the potential for a similar event happening in Illinois. After the immediate upheaval from the attack began to subside, public health professionals across the United States began looking at how states and localities were prepared to respond to large-scale emergencies. What they found was not encouraging.

During the intervening years, public health professionals have moved aggressively to address the gaps in emergency preparation and disaster response. One approach has involved bringing new partners into the effort. The IDPH Division of Oral Health responded to this particular challenge by actively seeking out and forging new partnerships and by building on existing relationships to give oral health professionals a greater voice and a larger role in planning and implementing emergency response systems.

To understand the role dentists and dental hygienists can have in emergency response, it is first important to appreciate the skills and resources this group of professionals brings to the table. Dentists and dental hygienists have basic skills and abilities that allow them to function as partners with

* Corresponding author.

[1] Formerly Division of Oral Health, Illinois Department of Public Health, Office of Health Promotion, Springfield, IL.

E-mail address: julie.janssen@illinois.gov (J.A. Janssen).

0011-8532/07/$ - see front matter
doi:10.1016/j.cden.2007.06.009 *dental.theclinics.com*

other health care providers in responding to a disaster. Oral health resources in the form of well-equipped and supplied dental offices and clinics have the potential to provide additional facilities for use during an emergency. As licensed health care professionals, dentists and dental hygienists should feel a responsibility to act if a disaster should occur in their communities. In Illinois, including dentists and dental hygienists as front-line responders could add approximately 14,000 licensed professionals to the response system. This significant pool of experience and human capital makes oral health professionals a valuable part of public health's emergency response efforts.

Encouraging oral health professionals in Illinois to see themselves as important components of state and local emergency preparedness efforts has been a natural role for Division of Oral Health staff. It also fits well with the division's mission, which is to ensure that the people of Illinois have access to population-based interventions that prevent and reduce oral disease and promote oral health as integral to overall health. Taking a leadership role, the division has helped to successfully integrate oral health professionals into the emergency medical response system in Illinois by performing the following:

- Raising awareness
- Building needed partnerships
- Identifying and garnering resources
- Facilitating training, policy development, surveillance, and evaluation

What has been done

Although the state's first oral health plan did not address the role of dentists and dental hygienists in disaster response, it did provide Illinois with a dynamic roadmap by which to accomplish this goal. The plan's guidance in building an oral health infrastructure in the state and in establishing and extending partnerships has enabled Illinois to initiate and maintain an exemplary oral health component in its overall disaster response program. But how did the state get to this point?

In 2002, Dr. Lewis Lampiris, then chief of the Division of Oral Health, participated in a consensus workshop sponsored by the American Dental Association (ADA). The workshop, entitled "The Role of Dentistry in Bioterrorism," helped to bring Illinois to the forefront of national response efforts by the ADA and other national groups. It also established an important working partnership between Illinois and the ADA that persists today.

During the summer of 2003, the division worked with Dr. Michael Colvard to establish the Disaster Emergency Medicine Readiness Training (DEMRT) Center at the University of Illinois at Chicago. In addition, Dr. Lampiris helped to secure funding for DEMRT through the IDPH's Office of Preparedness and Response. IDPH resources of funding, a multidisciplinary workforce, and expertise are critical not only to fuel DEMRT's activities but also to cement oral health as an integral component of the public health response system. By linking various IDPH divisions to DEMRT, an important new partnership was forged. DEMRT began to recruit, train, and retain volunteer medical responders, among them oral health professionals, who would be able to participate on local, state, or federal response teams. DEMRT provides the state surveillance and evaluation data that translates into information describing a successful program. This information is shared with a wide national audience as a model to help build similar efforts through out the United States. DEMRT provides a linkage not only between the IDPH and the University of Illinois and its College of Dentistry but also to associated professional organizations, such as the American Medical Association and a myriad of federal agencies, including the US Public Health Service.

In collaboration with DEMRT and the Illinois State Dental Society, the division began working in 2004 to expand the capacity to educate Illinois dentists and dental hygienists about the importance of emergency response preparation and to create training programs for dental responders at the local level. The division also helped to link oral health programs in local health departments to DEMRT to enable them to build training opportunities for dentists and dental hygienists, both in public and private practices, into community preparedness efforts.

In May 2005, the Division of Oral Health facilitated a satellite broadcast for dentists and dental hygienists in Illinois. The program, entitled "Disaster Preparedness: The Dental Team's Role," was planned and co-sponsored by DEMRT, IDPH, the Illinois State Dental Society, and the Illinois Dental Hygienists' Association. The presentations were designed to help the participants understand public health and preparedness efforts at the state and local level and how dentists and dental hygienists could become important partners. The IDPH Training Center arranged for 28 broadcast sites around the state. At each site, a Division of Oral Health staff person or other trained facilitator hosted the event and managed post-broadcast discussions.

The program brought together a panel of local, state, and national leaders in oral health and emergency preparedness. Response to the program was very positive. Participants indicated they understood their role in emergency response. They also were positive about seeking additional training and reaching out to the emergency response systems in their communities.

Another collaborative effort undertaken in 2005 by IDPH, DEMRT, and the Illinois State Dental Society effectively validated the role of dentists and dental hygienists in emergency response. Advocacy efforts by the group led to the amendment of the Illinois Dental Practice Act (P.A. 94-0409 25/4 Section 4[r]). As of December 31 that year, a "dental emergency responder" was defined as a dentist or dental hygienist appropriately certified in emergency medical response (as determined by the Illinois Department of

Public Health). The act was further amended to allow a responder to practice within the bounds of his or her license when providing care during a declared emergency (P.A. 94-0409 25/54.2 Section 54.2).

In 2006, the Division of Oral Health helped to lead the state in expanding and refining its statewide oral health plan. Unlike the first plan, this document dedicated a significant amount of attention to emergency preparedness, thereby ensuring it a platform for ongoing policymaking and program development. As with the first plan, the division enlisted a broad constituency of state and local leaders, as well as those at the grass-roots level. All shared an intense interest in improving the oral health of all Illinoisans and in expanding the plan's scope to include emergency response. By engaging these diverse stakeholders in the planning process, the division has ensured a strong and effective base for future actions.

What is on the horizon

Looking ahead, the division is involved on several fronts that promise to enhance the connection between oral health and emergency response in Illinois.

Expanding interdepartmental relationships

Within IDPH, the division is focusing on developing a closer working relationship with the Office of Preparedness and Response to expand communication between oral health professionals and community-based emergency response systems. It is equally critical for oral health professionals to understand and assume an appropriate role in disaster response as it is for community response systems to understand the value of including oral health professionals as partners in planning and training and in response when necessary.

As the state's oral health program, the division is positioned perfectly to accomplish this task. For more than 30 years, the division has placed staff in IDPH regional offices. These regional oral health consultants, who act as liaisons between the division and local health agencies, are adept at connecting community-level programs to state-of-the-art public health initiatives. For example, regional oral health consultants work with local staff to promote and implement programs such as community water fluoridation, oral health needs assessment and planning, dental sealants, Project Mouthguard, and oral cancer prevention and control. These regional staff can work through these existing relationships to promote partnerships with local emergency response efforts.

Oral health plan promotion

The division plans to continue its commitment to promote the state's oral health plan. As revised in 2006, the plan now includes an emergency preparedness and response component as a cornerstone of the state's oral health endeavors. The Illinois Oral Health Plan is widely distributed by the statewide oral health coalition, IFLOSS: Communities Working Together to Improve Oral Health in Illinois. Embracing the use of the Plan as the definitive planning and evaluation tool guiding local and state oral health improvement activities is a mission of the IFLOSS membership who include a broad public-private constituency. The IFLOSS coalition was instrumental in coordinating the state effort to create the state oral health plan and subsequently ensuring that it and all of the elements in it were implemented.

Policy development

The Division of Oral Health identifies opportunities for systemic, socio-political, and policy changes to improve oral health. Within the emergency response arena, the division will continue to help lead the state in policy development by working with primary stakeholders to define and implement the terms for dental emergency responder certification as dictated in the amended Illinois Dental Practice Act. The division will also assess the need for further policy changes to ensure that communities are prepared to use the services of dental emergency responders.

Stakeholder engagement

The division understands the critical importance of developing good working partnerships with many and varied stakeholders. To accomplish this, division staff continually scan the environment for opportunities to make contact with agencies and organizations involved in promoting oral health, particularly those that are working to enhance the connection between oral health professionals and those in emergency preparedness and response. Such contact provides important platforms for positive interaction.

Expanded capabilities

To expand its evaluation capabilities, the Division of Oral Health has added an epidemiologist to its staff. The addition provides the division with the skills, ability, and experience to create a tracking system that can monitor and evaluate progress toward the goal of integrating oral health professionals into the emergency medical response system. These evaluation activities should generate important data about such integration, data division leaders are committed to sharing with peers and partners throughout the United States. This continues a rich history of excellence for IDPH's Division of Oral Health, especially in the implementation and sharing of best practice models.

Applying the same principals and standards to the integration of oral health and disaster preparedness and response as it does to all facets of dental public health, the division will continue to cultivate its emerging leadership role. By continuing its efforts to raise awareness, to build needed partnerships, to identify and garner resources, and to facilitate training, policy development, surveillance, and evaluation, the division will reach and surpass its goal of integrating oral health professionals into the emergency medical response system in Illinois.

ELSEVIER
SAUNDERS

Dent Clin N Am 51 (2007) 785–803

THE DENTAL CLINICS OF NORTH AMERICA

The Importance of a Shared Vision in Emergency Preparedness: Engaging Partners in a Home-Rule State

Samuel Watson-Alván, MS,
Joseli Alves-Dunkerson, DDS, MPH, MBA*

Olympia, WA, USA

September 11, 2001 and Hurricane Katrina are experiences that touched all Americans. These events brought the need for effective emergency response to the forefront and exemplified what it takes to succeed and how easy it can be to fail.

> "Today there is a national consensus that we must be better prepared to respond to events like Hurricane Katrina. While we have constructed a system that effectively handles the demands of routine, limited natural and man-made disasters, our system clearly has structural flaws for addressing catastrophic incidents" [1].

Sharing a vision and spreading a culture of emergency preparedness to all levels of society is considered a national need and obsession. Obstacles exist, however, on the road to making it happen, some of which are inherent to human nature. For example, most human beings tend to forget the initial feelings of helplessness and frustration that a catastrophic event brings, giving place to more passive feelings of sorrow and remembrances. For people who face the issue and want to become active members of preparedness efforts, it can be overwhelming to decide how to do it, and inertia eventually kicks in. These are common coping mechanisms, not only of single individuals but also of communities and organizations. For emergency preparedness to be successful, anything less than an active approach allows history to repeat itself. For this reason, a powerful vision and a strong culture become essential tools for engaging partners and communities into the emergency preparedness movement. An overall challenge requires an overall response.

* Corresponding author. 2448 Boulevard Heights Loop SE, Olympia, WA 98501.
E-mail address: joseliad@comcast.net (J. Alves-Dunkerson).

0011-8532/07/$ - see front matter
doi:10.1016/j.cden.2007.06.007 *dental.theclinics.com*

> "...But we as a Nation—Federal, State, and local governments; the private sector; as well as communities and individual citizens—have not developed a shared vision of or commitment to preparedness: what we must do to prevent (when possible), protect against, respond to, and recover from the next catastrophe. Without a shared vision that is acted upon by all levels of our Nation and encompasses the full range of our preparedness and response capabilities, we will not achieve a truly transformational national state of preparedness. There are two immediate priorities for this transformation or change process: 1) to define (a vision for) and implement a comprehensive National Preparedness System; and 2) to foster a new, robust Culture of Preparedness" [1].

Defining vision and culture

A vision is an attempt to articulate a desired future. It identifies the end state we are seeking to achieve and how we plan to get there. It identifies core values and beliefs, is idealistic, inspiring, desirable, future oriented, bold and ambitious, unique, well articulated, and easily understood, and it represents broad and overarching goals. A well-articulated vision sets the horizon for the work to be done. Culture is a more elusive concept to define. Historically, cultures have emerged around a proposal for a vision that is embraced and held in sacred status by a collective. A culture can be recognized as the body and codification of symbols through which a community engages the projects of world building and meaning making. It provides the framework for processing information, developing knowledge, seeking awareness, and forming identity and relationships.

> "National preparedness involves a continuous cycle of activity to develop the elements (eg, plans, procedures, policies, training, and equipment) necessary to maximize the capability to prevent, protect against, respond to, and recover from domestic incidents, especially major events that require coordination among an appropriate combination of Federal, State, local, tribal, private sector, and non governmental entities, with the goal of minimizing the impact on lives, property, and the economy" [1].

The challenge ahead is how to share such vision successfully at the state and local levels, within public health, other government, and nonprofit and private sectors and how to do it in a way that not only is compatible with and attractive to the local reality but also formulates a strengthened and more contemporary public health culture.

The growing role of public health

Although the emergency preparedness movement is multisectorial (Fig. 1), public health agencies are viewed as one of the cornerstones of emergency preparedness programs. This role has evolved historically more out of necessity than appropriate planning. Already in 1988, the Institute

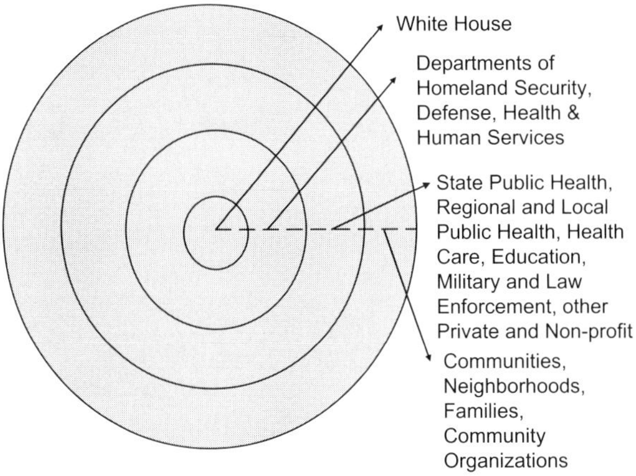

Fig. 1. Multisectorial response model.

of Medicine (IOM) published a scathing report entitled "The Future of Public Health" [2]. This study was undertaken to "address a growing perception among the IOM membership and others concerned with the health of the public that this nation has lost sight of its public health goals and allowed the system of public health activities to fall in disarray."

At a time when the traditional problems that gave birth to public health seemed to have been conquered by the escalating successes of science and not a few pharmaceutical "miracles," the IOM turned its attention to public health as a social service field and analyzed its deficiencies as such. This IOM report was visionary and established organizational and programmatic models for public health that were considered at the time contemporary and innovative in the highest sense of these words. The IOM report even went so far as to note the need to successfully counter continuing and emerging public health threats. Its listing of such threats, however, was limited by the times and unable to foretell events of the magnitude of those that occurred on September 11, 2001 and thereafter, including the 2006 Gulf storms, the looming threat of a deadly influenza pandemic, and the emergence of drug-resistant diseases such as tuberculosis.

From the limits of its vantage point, IOM members forged a vision for public health based on the government's mission of ensuring social conditions in which people can be healthy, which still guides public health activities. The core functions under that mission were listed as "assessment, policy development, and assurance." The limits of this awareness in effect sealed public health's retreat from the trenches into the sanctuary of social programs based on prevention activities. At no time did the IOM membership recognize that unforeseen future circumstances would propel public health back into the trenches, revealing more clearly than ever before its archetypical function as an emergency response capacity during emergencies and disasters of every ilk.

A second report from IOM, "The Future of the Public's Health in the 21st Century," which was released in 2002, expanded the initial framework [3]. More keenly focused on the largess of future challenges rather than the successes of the field, the report strongly propounded on the need for and value of multisectorial engagement in overcoming them. In a remarkable post-9/11 state of awareness, IOM stated that public health alone (ie, government and its traditional partners in that endeavor) were no longer sufficient to confront the current reality of what it would take to promote and protect the health of the population in the twenty-first century. More than ever, these suggestions hold true for the field of public health preparedness and response.

The report made only passing reference to the challenges of getting public health ready to confront a large complex and fluid emergency, such as pandemic flu, although it did agree that among six paramount action areas two would be to strengthen governmental public health infrastructure and develop a multisectorial public health system based on more robust partnerships with the public health system, the community, the health care delivery system, employers and business, the media, and academia.

Overall federal, state, and local public health efforts

After the events of September 11, 2001, the Bush administration communicated to the public health community a sense of urgency to plan for the likelihood of a terrorist attack involving weaponized smallpox virus. The underlying vision was not clear then, and even currently there is still scant evidence of its intent. Although the public health community remained skeptical overall, health departments around the nation set to work on the challenge of emergency preparedness and response planning around this potential hazard. Federal funding was allocated to states with strict requirements for response plans, along with hard and fast deadlines bordering on the unreasonable.

For individuals who were involved in these efforts, it soon became evident that public health peers, other government functionaries, and potential partners whose primary preoccupation was to administer public health programs under the faithful model suggested by IOM in 1988 held a different set of priorities. The threat, many argued, was not credible enough and was largely considered political hype. A generalized attitude of guarded collaboration sent a clear message to emergency preparedness professionals that the public health community's broad belief was that "this too shall pass" and public health would get back to its business of running prevention and regulatory programs soon enough. Many states and local health departments initially refused to change their organizational structures to accommodate preparedness programs, placing them as an add-on or as a special and temporary function—like a burden on a system that refused to accept that the world had changed—to accept funds that would help rebuild an otherwise neglected public health infrastructure under the guise of emergency preparedness.

The willingness of the federal government to provide copious funding for emergency preparedness to states and local jurisdictions, public health leaders argued, was precisely that: an opportunity to capitalize on and get public health on the political radar screen so that the "real" work of public health might be known by all and resourced as deserved. In effect, the national vision for public health as the social service field of the 1980s remained basically unchanged and unable to accommodate the awareness that a new era had begun with the new millennium. For several reasons, the nation, if not the world, had to function in an environment of quickly evolving threats, any of which could overwhelm existing response systems and their current levels of preparedness at any given time, and at the time public health suffered from a large scotoma about the full implications for its role in that environment.

In many cases, the public health community continues to struggle with that vision impairment. Public health program managers and staff have difficulty seeing the relevance of emergency preparedness to their scope of work; collaboration is limited by competing priorities and, in some instances, is contentious. Training and cross-training of public health professionals for the sake of creating a robust system of response based on redundancies and staffing schemes with bench strength and depth has been painfully slow. The involvement of external partners to bolster surge, supplemental capacity also has been paused, particularly outside of the more traditional cadre of players, and it remains distant from constituting a "system."

Despite these difficulties, much and laudable work has been accomplished at the federal, state, and local levels in the span of 5 years. Beyond any argument, the national public health system continues to change in significant ways and is better prepared than ever to understand its potential challenges.

The Washington State scenario

The Evergreen State has been in the process of developing its public health emergency preparedness and response program since 2002 [4]. A brief analysis of this program follows based on Kotter's [5] framework on successful change management.

Establishing a sense of urgency: state's threat assessment

There is little room for doubt that Washington State is territory primed to experience the potentially catastrophic effects of natural disasters and perhaps other types of emergencies with a public health dimension [6]. Washington is a land of telluric forces—natural, social, political, economic—that create conditions favorable to disasters and other emergencies involving massive losses and casualties, and with a potential to overwhelm the capacity of the health system to deal with them at any given time.

In Washington's modern history hardly a year has gone by when there was not either a major federal disaster or emergency declaration or a significant fire management assistance declaration. Besides storms, flooding, tidal surges, and landslides, in the last 40 years the state has experienced a volcano eruption of global scale (Mount Saint Helen), four major earthquakes in modern times (1872 in the Cascade Mountains, 1949 in Olympia, 1965 in Bremerton, and 2001 in Olympia), a major drought, and several catastrophic wildfires. More similar events are prognosticated and likely to continue to occur with some increase in frequency, larger impact, or both.

Adding to Washington's proclivity for natural disasters is the country's current political positioning in a global environment of growing discontent with US foreign policy. These circumstances have laid a context for multiple threats, thwarted attempts against visible targets, and actual attacks against the nation. Within Washington's boundaries are found ports of entry with international prominence and high traffic volume and target value. The city of Seattle, the state's financial center, continues to increase its gravitational pull on the national and international tourism industry, global financial markets, and international commerce of every sort partly because of its highly visible industries, aesthetic beauty, benign climate, and strategic location—features that also make the city highly vulnerable. When added up, these factors significantly elevate Washington's threat vulnerability coefficient regarding intentional acts of disruption and attacks of every sort (eg, chemical, biologic, radioactive).

A read of the evolving threat environment discloses that the occurrence of emerging and drug-resistant diseases, vector borne/zoonotic diseases, and other public health threats tied to environmental factors is on the rise around the world. Climate change, increased global commerce, demographic explosion, changes in species migration patterns, mass food production, and processing strategies are creating fertile conditions for the threat of infectious and communicable diseases to increase significantly in the foreseeable future. Many of these disease outbreaks tend to originate in densely populated and poorly sanitized third world countries with which Washington maintains prolific commercial ties. During the 2004 SARS outbreaks, the Washington public health community had to respond to one such threat and is currently undergoing intense preparations against a potential outbreak of pandemic influenza given the state's role as a portal to the high volume markets of the Far East. Sea-Tac Airport also is the designated diversion airport for the West Coast to where any flight transporting refugees, criminal acts in progress, or ill and diseased passengers will be directed.

There is no way of knowing which, if any, of these threats will take place in Washington in the near future. There is no doubt, however, that the potential for something to happen on a scale that would impose a significant deployment of available health-related resources is present at any time. Such a scenario would require the capacity to maximize the potential of the public health system, including imaginative use of alternative or supplemental resources to cover any surge demands in current capacity. It also challenges the Washington public health community to engage the project of broadening its vision and building a culture of public health readiness without delay.

The effective deployment of a system for surge capacity under emergency conditions demands that a great deal of infrastructure development and preparedness measures be in place before the occurrence of an event. To be sure, a sufficient canon of legislation exists in Washington to provide the Governor of the state and the Secretary of Health with enough authority to press into service any professional with a modicum of medical training and basic health care sense. It is not an unlikely picture to imagine, for example, dental professionals giving shots, operating ventilators, leading triage units, assessing vital signs, and even performing surgery as might be required by the situation and as their training allows.

Forming a powerful guiding coalition of partners: the heightened importance of partnerships in a home rule state

Washington State's home rule tradition

Washington State is known for its numerous coalitions and partnerships involving state and local governments and communities, especially those related to public health issues. This is a consequence of the strong expression of the "home rule" tradition in our state, which favors decentralized government and has been in place since 1948 (Article XI, § 4 of the Washington State constitution) [7,8]

The history of the State of Washington has been shaped by a combination of great events and movements, the settlement patterns described by a diverse population as communities formed across a geographically diverse territory, and the ways in which those communities chose to deal with historic events based on their local experience of place [9]

The coming of the railroad, populism, prohibition, municipal tax reform, public power, the Great Depression, property tax limitations, federal government assistance, and the great wars were historical benchmarks in the dialog that shaped the state's home rule tradition. Of no lesser significance was the physical and cultural isolation of early settlements along the lines of economic interest, ethnicities, and the exploitation of natural resources. Above all, the fiercely independent frontier spirit of pioneer Washingtonians helped determine how the political dialog on the issues evolved around values of self-determination, community, and participatory civil society.

Although not a true "home rule" in the legal sense, the strong culture of local governance and control in Washington is defined by two overarching characteristics: insistence on local option and control, including how state policy is shaped and implemented, and the unique relationship between local governance authorities, including special purpose districts authorized to provide specific services to the population, such as is the case of local health jurisdictions.

Over time, these relationships evolved to become more functional according to the issues of the time while all along reaffirming the underpinnings of the tradition of local control. Currently, these relationships are mostly defined by the prominent effects of growing fiscal pressures, population growth, environmental constraints of various kinds, and the need for equitable distribution and availability of services across the state. Inasmuch as Washingtonians tend to like local solutions to their problems, they want to be in charge of them and they want them to work well, perhaps better than those of their neighbors. Although through these efforts local governance relationships and traditions have evolved through time, however, they have not been able to keep pace with the speed and complexity of change in Washington, particularly in the last 60 years since World War II.

This is certainly the case in terms of the advent of a domestic security culture largely based on public health threats and concerns arising from the events of September 11, 2001, threats that—should they become reality—would be completely indifferent to geopolitical boundaries and the types of local concerns that dictate political protocol and policy development and implementation in Washington territory. For certain, these are threats whose potential is vastly more complex and exacting than the governance system's current design might be able to effectively deal with.

The public health perspective for how to engage the requisite preparations to respond to an attack to the homeland or, more currently, a pandemic event has been, predictably, to improvise on the existing system of local authority while causing minimal disruption of local politics and local-to-local and state-to-local governance relationships. The implications of these decisions for public health are significant and began in 2002 with the challenges involved in negotiating an adequate and equitable funding formula for 35 local health jurisdictions with variegated needs, challenges, threat vulnerabilities, and capabilities. Advantageously, the system that emerged, rightly or not, minimized the role of the state as a responder and placed the brunt of the responsibility on local jurisdictions.

The funding requirements for the state included ensuring a coordinated system of preparedness and response across jurisdictions based on such features as articulated plans, mutual aid, shared capacities, interoperable communications, coordinated risk management, and training standards. To fulfill its responsibilities, the state, in partnership with local health officials, instituted an extra-official reorganization of local health jurisdictions into nine "Public Health Emergency Planning Regions" (Fig. 2) responsible for the coordination of regional preparedness and response plans based on local plans and for the fiscal management of pass-through federal funds [10]. So far this system has sufficed for the timely production of the deliverables tied to that funding—if not for effective planning—and recently Washington was evaluated by Trust in America's Health, with high scores in

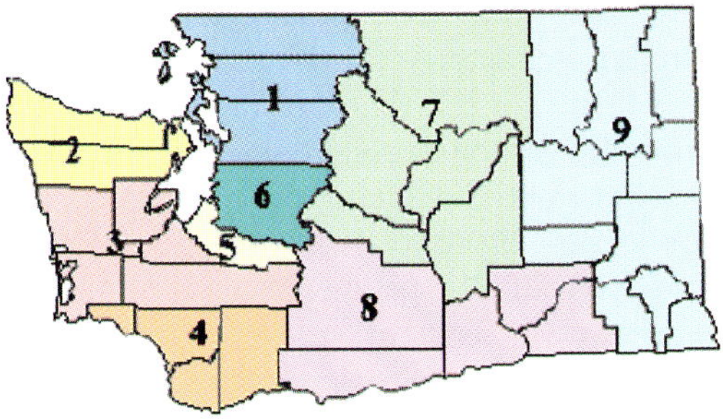

Fig. 2. Washington State's regional approach encourages coordination and resource sharing. At the local level, 39 counties are organized into 35 local health jurisdictions, which in turn come together as nine public health emergency planning regions. Local health jurisdictions' efforts on local emergency preparedness vary significantly, although they should be aligned at the regional level and with other community partners.

preparedness for bioterrorism, pandemic flu, and health disasters on that basis [11].

It is worthwhile remarking that the state's regional system of public health preparedness means that each region is responsible for such things as multisectorial partnerships, surge capacity, conducting a response, identifying and organizing supplemental providers to strengthen that response as needed, and articulating their efforts and plans with health care and other sectors. Should the demands of an emergency grow beyond a region's capacity to address it, that region is de facto responsible for invoking mutual aid agreements or requesting help from the state. In turn, the state is obliged to coordinate aid from other regions, states, or the federal government as needed in what is eminently a supporting role. The rationale for this model was fairly well cast by the traditions of home rule and Washington's geopolitics and followed the inertia of existing and prescribed logic.

To be objective, it is an open question whether the regional model will be able to effectively measure up to general threats "whose potential is vastly more complex and exacting than the governance system's current design might be able to effectively deal with." Will the system work smoothly or at least effectively during an emergency, such as might be a serious pandemic, in which all regions, states, and neighboring countries might suddenly find themselves competing for the same resources during the same time period?

This scenario has yet to be fully and realistically exercised at the statewide level. That is, the development of an exercise based on sound computer modeling that relies on what is currently known about the most likely virus with pandemic potential (H5N1) and tests for various outcomes has not yet made the work agenda. This should not come as a surprise. As a planning scenario, pandemic flu daunts public health planners. Planners overall seem to find the task of designing such an exercise—let alone imagining the likelihood of having to respond to the real disease—overwhelming. It is, however, the best known way to test the regional system outside of a real emergency with similar characteristics.

In the meantime, there is much that the state can and has left to do with regard to optimizing the response potential of local/regional public health partnerships. Its responsibilities and latitude for action are, however, limited by the collegial politics of local control and the tacit protocols defining those partnerships. Partnerships of all types can be a mixed blessing when it comes to undertaking work with a sense of urgency. Partnerships demand more time, resources, patience, and the wisdom of shared leadership. The demands of doing the work of partnership development often compete with the established priorities of reaching perceived goals and objectives expediently. Until Washington's public health preparedness and response partnerships are truly tested in a large-scale emergency, it remains to be seen whether the benefits of that work will have outweighed the pains. Currently, it remains a calculated risk.

It is broadly accepted that no better models currently exist for the purpose of optimizing response potential, at least in theory, than those that rely on a broad partnership base. Broadly speaking, this is not at issue in the Washington public health community with its inclination for participatory leadership. Regardless of what the effectiveness under fire of the regional system proves to be in the end, over time the state can be reasonably expected to do a better job of recognizing and optimizing the response potential of partnerships than other states with conflicting or less democratic traditions.

The state public health emergency preparedness and response program

Early in 2002, the federal government opened up two primary funding streams for public health preparedness. The first, through the Centers for Disease Control and Prevention, provided the greater part of the funds via a preparedness planning and infrastructure development grant. The second, through the Health Resources and Services Administration, provided considerably lesser funds to promote preparedness planning and infrastructure development in the health care sector. In Washington, both of these grants were administered by the Washington State Department of Health. These funding streams essentially represented two strong driving forces toward defining Washington's initial thrust for focusing on preparedness-based partnerships.

The Centers for Disease Control and Prevention grant required the department of health to work with local health jurisdictions, and the Washington State Association of Local Public Health Officers to develop public health capacity for emergencies. These partnerships had to evolve within the constraints and specificities of the state's geopolitical context.

The involvement of health organizations

Although the Centers for Disease Control and Prevention grant focused on developing a relationship with local health jurisdictions, the Health

Resources and Services Administration grant was designed to enhance the ability of hospitals and health care systems to be prepared for and respond to public health emergencies by supporting the development of bed and personnel surge capacity, decontamination capabilities, isolation capacity, pharmaceutical supplies, and supporting training, education, and drills and exercises. To implement this mandate, the department of health needed to seek partnerships with the health care sector, represented primarily by the Washington State Hospital Association. The department of health partnerships with the Washington State Hospital Association and the health care systems were forged painstakingly through careful discussions about best use of funds and a difficult sorting out of legal nuances regarding liability and compensation issues. The initial activities included a thorough assessment of hospital capacity in Washington State and the creation of communication systems to coordinate that capacity statewide.

Eventually, these partnerships expanded, consistent with the Health Resources and Services Administration's funding intent, to include stakeholders such as emergency medical services, tribes, community and migrant health clinics, home health care, poison control centers, and others. The state continues an active role of exploring the response potential of these partnerships.

Creating or recreating a vision

The salient question is whether the current public health system and its partners will be ready to respond to its potential challenges in rapid and fluid ways that capitalize on its every strength. Any potential answer to that question is certainly not as interesting or accessible as the question itself, a question that public health leaders must constantly ask of themselves and of those they lead. Any self-respecting strategist would agree that the work of being ready to hastily convene, morph, and deploy a system in several alternative ways as might be required by the fluid characteristics of a large complex emergency would be made easier if the vision guiding that leadership, its strategies, and the resources nurtured long before the emergency matches the requirements of the potential challenges.

For this reason, a vision for public health that recognizes public health's central role in emergencies and disasters would facilitate the early development of a public health culture that looks toward fulfilling this responsibility. That is, public health and its partners sorely need a generalized culture that provides them with an orientation for being ready and with the competencies to back it up regardless of its state of preparedness or prior knowledge of the emergency. A new public health culture that includes emergency preparedness and response as a core function must emphasize a constant state of readiness at the heart of its mission for ensuring conditions in which people can be healthy. Such a culture would have to be designed carefully, marketed emphatically, and nurtured incessantly if it were to replace the narrower public health culture of the 1980s before the next disaster strikes. These efforts should not be limited to public health professionals but extended to all potential partners and stakeholders in the success of the public health system.

Optimally, these efforts would include the promotion of a shared understanding for at least the following concepts:

- The certainty of future catastrophes
- The need for a constantly evolving state of readiness in an environment of fluid and emerging threats
- The importance of initiative and distributed social responsibility and leadership for proactive and fluid responses to large-scale emergencies
- The roles of each level of government, citizens, the private sector, and other stakeholders in public health, particularly in multi-hazard preparedness
- The roles of each of the health professions (including dentists and dental hygienists) with potential to become supplemental responders and health care providers at a time of crisis

The continuing transformation of the public health system is not solely a choice but an absolute necessity and a pressing leadership challenge. The dialog for the cultural transformation of public health first must be to establish reasonable expectations of what the government can and cannot do in response to catastrophes. Citizens should know what to expect from their government to make sure that they do everything possible at their level to protect themselves and their loved ones. Other sectors and stakeholders must likewise come to a better understanding of their growing scope of social responsibility in the preservation of the public health and civil society in general.

Communicating the vision

The renewed vision must be communicated through a marketing campaign that reaches all stakeholders, including the common person of every community. Otherwise, no vision will be powerful enough to help develop a system that meets the demands of a large-scale emergency that overwhelms government systems and other institutional support. It is worth noting that such an effort would be considerably expensive in a fiscal environment of thinly stretched government resources.

Empowering others to act on the vision: the involvement of health care professionals

If in the end Washington's model does not work as well as expected, it will certainly not be because the state, as the collection of multisectorial partnerships, in any way has refused to work together. Although many relationships remain to be formed or are still on the ground floor, the value of partnerships of all types is by and large well understood and practiced in Washington. Even so, in the best of cases, disaster scale emergencies can quickly overwhelm the response capacity of formal response systems and impose on them what is commonly referred to in the preparedness field as "surge demands."

Surge demands may be understood as spikes in the volume of requirements on a market or system that exceed said system's designed capacity to satisfy daily volume requirements on a routine basis. In the case of public health emergencies, surge demands can be expected to be sustained enough to require capacity to meet those surges beyond the response systems' stress limits. The redundancies and alternative design features that allow a system to face off with sustained surge demands is what public health is or should be concerned about. What is problematic is that how a specific surge capacity is defined vis-à-vis a specific demand dictates how resources are designed and allocated to the system. Miss the mark on defining surge capacity in relationship to demand, and the system may be designed with surge capacity but not necessarily of the kind and application that will satisfy the requirements of a particular event at any given time.

To explain further, if a hospital defines its surge capacity as the number of beds only, it might miss altogether addressing the requirements imposed by the volume of trauma patients arriving at the emergency room, along with the worried well family members who also require some aspect of support. One of the questions for defining surge capacity in this example might depend on measuring work flow speed versus patient volume in the emergency room. The definition of surge capacity is specific and relative to the resources in question and interdependent with the specificities of the demand for which that capacity is being designed. This analysis begs the questions of not simply adding more resources to a system to bolster surge capacity where evident but of what resources to add, how, where and when to add them, and for what specific reasons. Looked at from a perspective of complexity, designing for surge capacity becomes a careful game of strategy and not solely of numbers.

To address potential surge demands on public health and the capacity to meet them, in 2002 the federal government tied reporting mechanisms to funding for states and required them to describe their surge capacity to meet federally defined health care baselines by population size. In 2005 the Health Resources and Services Administration also released a program designed to fund an Emergency System for Advance Registration of Volunteer Health Professionals (ESARVHP). The guidance for ESARVHP stated that the system would be "an electronic database of health care personnel who volunteer to provide aid in an emergency." It would have to be capable of registering health volunteers, applying emergency credentialing standards to registered volunteers, and allowing for the verification of the identity, credentials, and qualifications of registered volunteers in an emergency. The federal guidance defined "health volunteer" as a medical or health care professional who renders aid or performs health services voluntarily without pay or remuneration.

The ESARVHP program required participating states to develop said databases following prespecified compliance standards that would allow for information exchange and coordination activities to take place between local jurisdictions and local-to-state, state-to-state, and state-to-federal relationships and culminate in the formation of a national network for volunteer coordination. In its next and final phase the program will require states to expand their systems to include credentialing standards for the following high-priority occupations:

- Advanced practice nurses (nurse practitioners, nurse anesthetists, certified nurse midwives, clinical nurse specialists)
- Physician assistants
- Dentists
- Dental hygienists
- Emergency medical technicians and paramedics
- Pharmacists
- Licensed practical nurses
- Respiratory therapists
- Respiratory therapy technicians
- Cardiovascular technologists and technicians
- Radiologic technologists and technicians
- Surgical technologists
- Medical and clinical laboratory technologists
- Medical and clinical laboratory technicians (including phlebotomists)
- Diagnostic medical sonographers
- Veterinarians

The State of Washington has been a participant in ESARVHP since its inception, although implementation has proceeded slowly and in a deliberate manner. The implications around the creation of a system of this type are of major significance to existing credentialing and professional regulatory state programs. There are political, legal, logistical, and resource issues to contend with over the long-term that are not easily unraveled and sorted out with the necessary foresight. As things frequently tend to go, federal requirements continue to be moving targets that have forced states to adapt on the go, sometimes causing delays in program development.

Currently, Washington has selected an ESARVHP vendor for an off-the-shelf system, called Washington Healthcare Volunteers in Emergencies (WAHVE), which is guaranteed to meet federal compliance standards as they evolve over time, with some room for customization. Initially, WAHVE will focus on implementing the first phase of ESARVHP only and it will be externally hosted and Web based, with features designed for resilience and a consumer-driven population of the database. Washington's participation in the program through WAHVE is a significant move that defines a policy direction committed to expanding the current base of professional partnerships related to emergency preparedness and response. Outreach work to professional associations, universities, and vocational colleges is to be expected in the future as part of the program's expansion and partnership development processes and will likely require additional allocation of resources to support the effort.

In these terms, Washington is doing as well as expected and keeping pace with federal requirements. The challenges of developing a system of surge capacity might go beyond adding up the numbers of beds, professionals, and professions available to do the work, however. The deeper work of strategically designing a system for surge capacity tied to specific demands that would cover a tapestry of hazards—and making that system effectively competent and deployable in various ways—has yet to be done. Much of that work resides on ensuring that the quality and scope of partnerships and the focus of the dialog driving the partnership development work, beyond the requirements of programs like ESARVHP, are consistent with the outstanding challenges.

The leadership responsibility for that work is the competence of all relevant and affected parties and not solely of state government. The extant strategic gaps and leadership challenges noted here are not a weakness limited to Washington but are inherent in the conceptual model currently practiced by government planners nationwide around the problem of addressing emergency surge demands in general and in the framework defining public expectations of what is the government's scope of responsibility in ensuring the health and safety of the public. The collective engagement in developing a system for surge capacity provides for an ideal imperative for optimizing the response potential of partnerships during public health emergencies.

As of December 2006, the number of licensed health care providers eligible for volunteering through WAHVE included 15, 758 physicians, 58,772 nurses, and 11,593 mental health care professionals. At least 5% of these professionals are expected to volunteer their services at WAHVE. The projected launch date for WAHVE is July 2007 for the first phase. It is important to remember that some local health departments (jurisdictions) already may have some type of local volunteer registry system in place by then. WAHVE aims at supporting local emergency preparedness efforts by creating a consistent tool to identify individuals statewide who want to volunteer, making this registry available to locals for identification of more volunteers, and facilitating the deployment of volunteers from out of state in case of larger disasters.

The involvement of the dental professions

A few states already have taken significant steps toward involving dental professionals in their emergency preparedness efforts [12–14]. In

Washington State, local oral health programs and dental professionals already have started to show interest in discussing their potential participation in emergency preparedness efforts. Several of the 35 local oral health programs already have been called to participate in their local emergency preparedness programs. Dental professionals are starting to brainstorm different forms of participation. Inclusion of dental professionals could lead to significant enhancement of the current emergency preparedness system, because in 2006, Washington State counted on 5648 licensed dentists and 4913 licensed dental hygienists [15]. Their professional expertise and office space could serve as important assets in terms of educating and protecting themselves, their families, their patients, and their neighbors.

The organizations that have shown interest in this initiative include the Washington State Dental Association, the Washington State Dental Hygienists' Association, the University of Washington School of Dentistry, and the eight dental hygiene programs. The Washington State Dental Association represents 3800 of the dentists and 189 dental hygienists in the state and counts on 19 local component societies. The Washington State Dental Association recently released a cover story discussing ways for dentists to provide help in case of disaster [16]. The Washington State Dental Hygienists' Association represents 1020 of the licensed dental hygienists in the state and counts on 14 local components. The University of Washington School of Dentistry graduates 55 students and the dental hygiene programs graduate 247 students per year. The concentration of dental professionals in urban areas may affect emergency response in rural areas.

Some concerns still exist about the participation of dental professionals in emergency preparedness: have they received specific EP training as other health care professionals? What would be the legal concerns regarding their action in EP? EP training exists at the local level, which helps to bring all volunteers to the same knowledge of how to work effectively as a team in an EP situation. The second question may be answered by two forms of legislation: SB 5054, which has extended off-limits the immunity of health professionals in cases of disasters [17], and HB 1850, which provides liability to retired volunteers in case of disasters [18].

While these partnerships evolve, one can gladly say that the collaborative mode in Washington is in good shape in terms of oral health. While the awareness is raised among dental partners, several steps are being planned for the near future, including

- Learning more about what other states are doing. For example, copies of the Illinois' DVD on disaster preparedness and the dental team have been distributed to local oral health programs and educational and professional associations.
- Finding ways to better integrate EP activities of the public and private sectors.

- Defining the different levels of interest demonstrated by dental professionals. For example, maxillofacial surgeons and military dentists may want to act as first responders, whereas other dental providers may not. It is important to note that in a disaster, most affected individuals need comforting and mental health counseling, not necessarily clinical procedures. Dental professionals also may have to deal with nonclinical issues.
- Identifying the existing skill level of dental providers that might be useful for primary or secondary responders, beyond dental identification (forensic dentistry).
- Developing an emergency preparedness curriculum for dental and dental hygiene students, and a continuing education module for seasoned dental professionals to raise their awareness to this matter. Some dental hygiene schools are already developing tentative emergency plans for dental providers and presenting them to local dental hygiene components.
- Making presentations on emergency preparedness throughout the state via local dental societies and state conferences.
- Participating in regular meetings with all interested partners.

Planning for and creating short-term wins

As the State of Washington moves forward with WAHVE, the partnership models that emerge from working with the cadre of stakeholders involved in the initial implementation phase will provide a base of experience for how to approach the challenges of expanding the database and developing a system for the coordination of supplemental providers during emergencies. Credentialing requirements may change. Training competencies and academic requirements may have to be revisited. Legal issues must be resolved. Not least of all, the value of professional associations and education institutions must be recognized not only as a source of additional resources but also an aid in furthering the public health vision for emergency readiness.

Consolidating improvements and producing more changes

In the end, it is through a comprehensive program of drills and exercises or during actual responses that the complete collection of response assets will "learn" to know itself and operate as a system. Strengthening the state's planning function to involve external stakeholders from all sectors in helping facilitate the learning curve is a major factor in the emergence of effective multisectorial response capacity.

Institutionalizing new approaches

Beyond all the hard work that public health and health care professionals and other responders will be called to do, nothing can guarantee success like the institutionalization of their partnerships under a common vision and operating culture. The arguments that have been presented in this article are supported by the IOM successes in establishing its social service vision for public health in the late 1980s and tracing the tremendous legacy of their landmark work "The Future of Public Health" 20 years past. It is time to take that work to its next level by putting emergency readiness in the crosshairs of a new multisectorial vision for public health.

Final thoughts

Although emergency preparedness efforts in Washington State are keeping pace with national requirements, it is clear that a broader vision and culture must be shared statewide, always respecting the state's home rule tradition. How a regionalized model will respond to a general threat remains to be seen. Although dental professionals are not currently included in the state's emergency preparedness program, the wheels have been put in motion to increase their awareness and involvement. Dental professionals are trained in a multitude of skills that could be useful to emergency response at different levels. The state's public health, professional, and educational organizations are currently starting to dialog about potential ways for involving dental professionals. It is safe to say that whatever happens, public health will continue its pathfinding work and Washington State will reach satisfying results.

Acknowledgments

This article would not have been possible without the contribution of the following individuals: Edmond L. Truelove, DMD, MSD, Chair and Professor of the Department of Oral Medicine at the University of Washington School of Dentistry; Rhonda Savage, DDS, President of the Washington State Dental Association; and Gene M. Patterson, MA, Executive Director of the Washington State Dental Hygienists' Association. Their willingness and ability to foresee and understand the value of the potential role of dental professionals in emergency preparedness were key to the writing of this article and will be a pivotal factor to the success of emergency preparedness efforts within the dental professions in Washington.

References

[1] The White House. Transforming national preparedness: the federal response to Hurricane Katrina. Lessons learned; 2006. Available at: http://www.whitehouse.gov/reports/katrina-lessons-learned. Accessed January 2007.

[2] Institute of Medicine, Committee for the Study of the Future of Public Health, Division of Health Care Services. The future of public health. Washington, DC: National Academy Press; 1988.

[3] Institute of Medicine, The Committee on Assuring the Health of the Public in the 21st Century. The future of the public's health in the 21st century. Washington, DC: National Academies of Press; 2002.
[4] Public Health Emergency Preparedness and Response Program. Available at: http://www.doh.wa.gov/phepr/default.htm. Accessed February 2007.
[5] Kotter JP. Leading change: why transformation efforts fail. Harv Bus Rev 1995;59–67.
[6] FEMA. Washington State disaster history. Available at: http://www.fema.gov/news/disasters_state.fema?id=53. Accessed December 2006.
[7] Does my state have home rule? Available at: http://www.celdf.org/HomeRule/DoesmyStatehaveHomeRule/tabid/115/Default.aspx. Accessed January 2007.
[8] Home rule in Washington State. Available at: http://www.celdf.org/HomeRule/DoesmyStatchaveHomeRule/HomeRuleinWashingtonState/tabid/157/Default.aspx. Accessed January, 2007.
[9] Washington State Local Government Study Commission. A history of Washington's local governments 1988. Available at: http://www.mrsc.org/govdocs/VolILocalGovHistory.pdf. Accessed February 2007.
[10] Washington State Department of Health. Washington State public health emergency preparedness and response: regions. Available at: http://www.doh.wa.gov/phepr/regions.htm. Accessed February 2007.
[11] Washington receives 8 out of 10 for bioterror, bird flu, and health disaster preparedness. Available at: http://healthyamericans.org/reports/bioterror06/release.php?StateID=WA. Accessed December 2006.
[12] Glotzer DL, Psoter WJ, Rekow ED. Emergency preparedness in the dental office. J Am Dent Assoc 2004;135(11):1565–70.
[13] Lopatin DE. Emergency preparedness: a new role for the dental practitioner. J Mich Dent Assoc 2004;86(12):24–8.
[14] Colvard MD, Lampiris LN, Cordell GA, et al. The dental emergency responder: expanding the scope of dental practice. J Am Dent Assoc 2006;137(4):468–73.
[15] Byrappagari D, Alves-Dunkerson JA, Chamie C, et al. The impact of oral disease on the lives of Washingtonians: the Washington State oral disease burden document. Olympia (WA): Washington State Department of Health; 2007.
[16] Washington State Dental Association. If a disaster strikes, how can you help? WSDA News 2007:20–2.
[17] Senate Bill 5054. Concerning limited emergency worker volunteer immunity, 2007–08. Available at: http://apps.leg.wa.gov/billinfo/summary.aspx?bill=5054&year=2007. Accessed March 2007.
[18] House Bill 1850. Creating a retired volunteer medical worker license, 2005–06. Available at: http://apps.leg.wa.gov/billinfo/summary.aspx?bill=1850&year=2005. Accessed March 2007.

ELSEVIER
SAUNDERS

Dent Clin N Am 51 (2007) 805–818

THE DENTAL CLINICS OF NORTH AMERICA

All Hazards Training: Incorporating a Catastrophe Preparedness Mindset into the Dental School Curriculum and Professional Practice

David L. Glotzer, DDS[a,*],
E. Dianne Rekow, PhD, DDS[b],
Frederick G. More, DDS, MS[c,d],
Benjamin Godder, DMD[a], Walter Psoter, DDS, PhD[c,e]

[a]*Department of Cariology and Comprehensive Care, New York University College of Dentistry, 423 E. 23rd Street, VA, 16N, New York, NY 10010, USA*
[b]*Department of Basic Science and Craniofacial Biology, New York University College of Dentistry, 345 E. 24th Street, New York, NY 10010-4086, USA*
[c]*Department of Epidemiology and Health Promotion, New York University College of Dentistry, 345 E. 24th Street, New York, NY 10010-4086, USA*
[d]*Department of Pediatric Dentistry, New York University College of Dentistry, 345 E. 24th Street, New York, NY 10010-4086, USA*
[e]*School of Dentistry, University of Puerto Rico, Puerto Rico*

The events of September 11, 2001 and the subsequent anthrax scare triggered an unprecedented concern for public health preparedness and uneasiness about the nation's capacity to defend itself against and respond to another terrorist attack. This awareness prompted the public health community to focus on ways to increase surge capacity by increasing the number of available and trained personnel to respond to mass casualty events. In early 2002, the leadership of the New York University College of Dentistry (NYUCD) sought to define a role for the dental profession in response to the new threats of terrorism the United States was facing. One initiative proposed expanding the dental school curriculum to include bioterrorism studies and training across the 4 years of dental education to prepare dentists to respond and contribute to a public health disaster.

In parallel, the American Dental Association began to focus on defining the role of dentists in responding to a bioterrorism attack. The specific areas

* Corresponding author.
E-mail address: dlg2@nyu.edu (D.L. Glotzer).

0011-8532/07/$ - see front matter
doi:10.1016/j.cden.2007.06.003

of concern were (1) what preparation was required to respond to an attack, including the appropriate role of dental schools in training dentists to respond and (2) to what extent, if any, training should be mandated. The outcome of a consensus meeting was that bioterrorism training should occur within the dental school predoctoral curriculum and that all dentists should receive at least a basic level of bioterrorism training, including training that would enable them to recognize diseases and provide treatment and preventive measures under the direction of a responsible emergency response agency [1].

The American Dental Association and the American Dental Education Association then cosponsored a workshop entitled "Terrorism and Mass Casualty Curriculum Development." Participants recommended that core competencies be taught to all dental students to familiarize them with the potential agents that might be used in an attack, prepare them to respond to a significant attack, and create a cadre of aware health care professionals who could serve as a source of surveillance information in the event of an attack. The workshop participants concluded that although the addition of new courses related to bioterrorism to the curriculum would allow for more extensive training, the already crowded predoctoral curriculum leaves little room for the addition of entirely new courses. A more realistic approach would be to incorporate materials to address the core competencies into existing courses [2].

Proposed updated American Dental Education Association guidelines for competencies of graduate dentists also include the ability to "develop a catastrophic preparedness plan for the dental office," a component of best practices that addresses the personal professional level response to a catastrophic event [3]. To achieve this goal, a minimal understanding of disaster agents/consequences/responses must be learned either through dental school training or continuing education. The knowledge and skills to meet this American Dental Education Association competency are immediately transferable to the dentists' and staffs' homes and families. With this new skill, dentists—respected community members—are positioned to positively influence the local response planning at the governmental, agency, and local organizational levels.

Private dental practice and dental educational institutions provide a community health care resource that has the potential to provide assistance to prevent, prepare, respond, and recover during a catastrophic event. A survey of dental and medical school deans and state dental society presidents demonstrated that key professional and educational leadership consider dentists to have skills that can be part of a disaster response; in fact, they have an ethical obligation to provide assistance during the response to such an event. To be effective, however, they agreed that some type of significant additional training and integration into an organized response system is needed [4]. Through existing, formal opportunities in advanced training and participation in organized responder systems, hospital-based and public health dentists are a particularly valuable potential pool of skilled persons who can fill important roles during a response.

Catastrophic preparedness education and training for dentists and dental personnel is based on predoctoral initial basic competencies, postdoctoral training competencies, elective continuing education, and special, advanced programs for some dentists. Table 1 outlines a concept of this training and educational spectrum. This article presents (1) how faculty become trained in catastrophe preparedness, (2) proposed predoctoral dental competencies, (3) an approach to integrating catastrophic event basic science issues into the dental school curriculum, (4) a description of the capstone catastrophe preparedness course, and (5) suggestions on postdoctoral training components, continuing education recommendations, and advanced responder opportunities for dentists.

Faculty involvement

One of the most important issues related to introducing catastrophic preparedness into the dental school curriculum was the necessary preparation and training of the dental faculty. New York City remains on one continuous post-9/11 alert; every day the people of New York City see heightened subway security with National Guard soldiers at the major train stations and heavily armed police at the bridges and tunnels. Add to the mix potential natural disasters and threats such as avian flu, and the concept of having to do more to prepare is never out of mind of a responsible health care professional.

Table 1
Catastrophic response education and training spectrum

Predoctoral	Postdoctoral	Continuing education	Advanced responder
Basic science integration	Basic medicine principles[a]	Basic science aspects	Community emergency response team
Office management	Basic surgical principles[a]	Office management	Medical reserve corps
Basics in catastrophic events	Basic trauma principles[a]	Basics in catastrophic events	National disaster medical systems
Core disaster life support	Principles of triage	Principles of triage	
	Advanced cardiac life support	Advanced cardiac life support	
	Basic disaster life support	Basic disaster life support	
	Institution disaster plan	National incident command system	
	National incident command system		
	Decontamination		

[a] Integrated with medical, surgical, and anesthesia training.

In response to the NYUCD dean's vision to define a role for the dental profession in the months after 9/11, faculty with varied backgrounds stepped forward. This group shared the willingness and a sense of duty to contribute in this national emergency. They were dentists who had backgrounds in microbiology, epidemiology, oral pathology, oral medicine, or general dentistry, and some—but not all—had military experience. The interested faculty developed their individual skills and knowledge as essential components toward achieving the goal of improved expertise within the college on matters related to bioterrorism. The development of the individual faculty members and the success and enthusiasm of the new program were linked together [5].

The curriculum goal was all hazards training: incorporating a multidisciplinary mindset into the dental school curriculum to enhance medical and public health capabilities during time of crisis when current response resources at the national and local level would likely be overwhelmed. The faculty members involved with the catastrophic preparedness development participated in a diverse set of activities to bring themselves and the group to a satisfactory level for curriculum development in all-hazards training. Several notable activities assisted in the process for training and curriculum development. First, an expert panel was established to standardize and certify faculty instructors for preparedness and disaster response training. The expert panel included eight dental faculty members, two oral and maxillofacial surgeons, two pediatric dentists, one oral medicine specialist, one general practitioner, and two additional with military command and chemical, biologic, radiologic, nuclear, and explosive expertise. Their objective was to set the standards.

Dental and medical school and nursing faculty attended comprehensive 5-day training courses at Fort Sam Houston in San Antonio, Texas. These courses were designed by the US Army's Nuclear, Biological and Chemical Sciences Division of the Army's Health Sciences School. The purpose of this training was to enhance the knowledge base regarding bioterrorism and weapons of mass destruction, including chemical, biologic, radiologic, nuclear, and explosive devices. The course also outlined the role of military dentists as triage officers on the battlefield, delineated the role of the government agencies in the chain of command, and engaged the participants in case seminars and a field exercise designed to enable the participants to experience setting up a decontamination station and effectively treating casualties in a simulated terrorist attack [6].

Three faculty pioneered and completed didactic and clinical training in mass casualties/biologic and chemical triage by participating in a series of courses conducted by the American Medical Association (AMA) on disaster life support from core through basic and advanced levels (core disaster life support [CDLS], basic disaster life support [BDLS], and advanced disaster life support [ADLS], respectively). These courses stressed a comprehensive all-hazards approach to help physicians and other health professionals deal with catastrophic emergencies from man-made acts and explosions, fires, natural disasters, and the outbreak of infectious diseases [7]. These faculty members are certified trainers able to conduct the CDLS and BDLS courses.

Under the direction of the New York City Department of Health, points of distribution (POD) exercises have been conducted at the NYUCD. In the case of a natural epidemic or bioterrorist attack, mass prophylaxis or vaccinations may be required. To dispense antibiotics or vaccine to the public, PODs would be set up, requiring thousands of health professionals as staff. In these PODs, clinic roles are assigned to each health professional based on his or her skills and licensure. Hundreds of NYUCD faculty and students participated, expanding the trained reserve [8].

Three faculty members participated in six disaster response seminars developed by NYU Medical School's emergency medicine faculty and participated in a mini-internship in the emergency medicine department at Bellevue Hospital where, under the direction of emergency room physicians, they were exposed to the skills of rapid patient evaluation and the search for underlying systemic disease [9]. Nine faculty members were trained by the New York Department of Health and Mental Hygiene in telephone triage for an avian flu outbreak. Five of these participants are currently part of New York City's Medical Reserve Corps (MRC) specifically assigned to the health department for telephone triage duties.

These dental faculty members became the core group of faculty instructors who currently teach undergraduate and postgraduate students and conduct continuing education courses that have enabled NYUCD to become a recognizable and accredited center for basic and advanced level of training in CDLS and BDLS.

Dental student competencies

There are predictable challenges to be addressed when developing curriculum for predoctoral students. One challenge is to accept that dental curricula are overcrowded with clock hours. Curriculum committees usually demand that something be cut when faculty propose new subjects. How do we add content that is viewed as essential within the context of the dental curriculum? A second challenge is to determine what content is appropriate to add. A third challenge is constructing content that is carefully integrated into curriculum. Developing competencies early in the process served as a template to develop specific content material that meets the needs of entry-level dentists regardless of where they practice.

A few assumptions guided us as we developed competencies for our predoctoral students: (1) Catastrophic events take different forms, none of which is predictable. (2) Most dentists are less likely to be first responders and more likely to be community resources in an integrated response. (3) Dentists, by virtue of their overall education, have skills that can be applied directly or adapted easily when needed. Integration within current instruction had to be the hallmark of any new education programs. (4) Dentists who were willing to be first responders would need additional education beyond their predoctoral education. (5) Dentists, as members of their community, would be accountable for developing personal protection plans to ensure their safety and survival so that they would remain community resources. (6) Dentists, regardless of their education, faced the ethical dilemma of deciding whether to join in their community's response or stand aside.

Based on these assumptions, we developed the following competencies for dental graduates [10]:

- Competency 1: Describe the potential role of dentists in the first/early response in a range of catastrophic events.
- Competency 2: Describe the chain of command in the national, state, and/or local response to a catastrophic event.
- Competency 3: Demonstrate the likely role of a dentist in an emergency response and participate in a simulation/drill.
- Competency 4: Demonstrate the possible role of a dentist in all communications at the level of a response team, the media, to the general public, and to patient and family.
- Competency 5: Identify personal limits as a potential responder and sources that are available for referral.
- Competency 6: Apply problem solving and flexible thinking to unusual challenges within the dentist's functional ability and evaluate the effectiveness of the actions that are taken.
- Competency 7: Recognize deviations from the norm, such as unusual cancellation patterns, symptoms of seasonal illnesses that occur out the normal season, and employee absences, that may indicate an emergency and describe appropriate action.

Catastrophic preparedness in the New York University College of Dentistry dental curriculum

NYUCD incorporated training into the existing curriculum and added a concluding capstone course in the senior year. The overall goals of the program, which we describe as "catastrophe preparedness" in keeping with the current US Department of Homeland Security concept of an "all hazards" approach to emergency planning and are in concert with the seven specific competencies, are that students should (1) recognize the indications of an event, (2) react to the acute needs of the victims of such an event, (3) be able to participate in an orderly coordinated response to an event, and (4) know how to alert the public health system and understand how it reacts on all levels of government to the event. New elements of the curriculum were integrated into existing curriculum to the maximum extent possible. New components are modular so they could be shared easily with other dental schools. An actively participating senior capstone course described later incorporates evaluation by means of a pre- and postcourse questionnaire. NYUCD has put into place a new experience for dental students. Specific elements of this experience and their distribution through the curriculum are summarized as follows [11].

Freshman curriculum (D1). Shelter in place, emergency evacuations, and fire hazard (as part of D1 orientation). Total additional time in D1: 1 hour

NYUCD has an extensive emergency plan and shelter-in-place protocol in effect. The college is prepared and has water, food, and blankets on hand to shelter 1000 individuals for 3 days. This plan and protocol is presented to incoming students. This presentation also stresses the need for everyone to have a personal emergency plan, a "go-pak" ready with needed emergency items, and references to Web sites (such as www.ready.gov), which provides complete and comprehensive individual and family preparedness planning information. Because most students are not from the New York City area, this information sensitizes them to living in a potential high-target region and the protective actions needed.

Sophomore curriculum (D2). Agents of bioterrorism: pathogens (as part of the general pathology and infectious diseases course). Total additional time in D2: 7 hours

In year two of the dental curriculum, the concept of inserting new modular elements into existing courses, with particular emphasis on the Centers for Disease Control and Prevention category "A" agents, is used. These bioagents can be disseminated easily or transmitted from person to person, result in high mortality rates and have the potential for major public health impact, might cause public panic and social disruption, and require special action for public health preparedness. The emphasis is on bacterial and viral entities and the toxins that comprise those agents, how they may be spread, how they are treated, and why a bioterrorist might select them.

Junior curriculum (D3). Oral and systemic manifestations of bioterrorist agents: Clinical signs and symptoms (as part of the course entitled "Care of the Medically Complex Patients"). Total additional time in D3: 3 hours

Students are introduced to oral and systemic manifestations of bioterrorist agents, including clinical signs and symptoms. Clinical symptoms of anthrax, smallpox, and plague are reviewed. Smallpox vaccine and possible complications are presented, and chemical agents, such as nerve, blood, and choking and blister agents, are introduced.

Senior curriculum (D4). Catastrophic preparedness course.
Total additional time in D4: 12 hours

Having experienced the total dental curriculum over their first 3 years, the senior year (D4) students have the basic foundation skills in the biomedical sciences, including biologic agents, an overview of chemical and biologic weapons, CPR training, and wound management and are well trained in infection control procedures. In their freshman year they also experienced the impact of an ethics course that explores a dentist's obligation to the community. The objective of the D4 course is to integrate their knowledge, and it culminates in students preparing an emergency plan for their own office [3].

Catastrophe preparedness course

After developing the modular educational content that was placed into existing courses, the faculty addressed the challenge of developing a stand-alone D4 program that would build on the curriculum components—together with the students' patient care and patient management experience—and integrate this knowledge into usable skills. These are some of the questions that had to be answered: What competencies should be reinforced? What instructional methods should be used (lecture, role play, seminars)? How should student attitudes and the course effectiveness be evaluated?

Because the fourth-year course was placed in the spring semester within 2 months of graduation, it was quickly determined that with the average student's state of mind at that time, the emergency preparedness course material had to be presented in a particularly effective, attention-getting manner. The first issue addressed is to reinforce why dentists should be concerned and be involved in catastrophic preparedness. This concept was considered of such critical importance that it is given in an introductory lecture delivered by the dean of the dental school. The lecture emphasizes to the students their obligation to the profession, the community, their own families, and the "flag." The lecture also elaborates to the students the skills they bring with them in the event of an emergency. The opportunities available to join an organized response effort, such as the MRC, are discussed [11].

The second theme of the course is the need to be part of and play a role in the community's established and organized disaster response system. The approach taken to achieve this objective is to demonstrate an existing public health surge response system. We capitalize on NYUCD's close relationship with the NYC Department of Health and Mental Hygiene. They provided us with their POD training materials. In an emergency, a POD could be established to distribute antibiotics or vaccinate populations quickly. It engages a multidisciplinary group of volunteer health professionals, including physicians, pharmacists, dentists, nurses and nurse practitioners, mental health practitioners, and others. Clinical/support roles are assigned to each professional based on their skills and licensure [12]. As part of the first course, students participated in a 3-hour POD drill with an improvised scenario, during which the NYUCD main auditorium was transformed into a smallpox vaccine dispensing center as our students acted as both members of the MRC (triaging, evaluating, dispensing, and inoculating the public) and as patients eagerly looking for protection. The exercise was filmed and can be used in future classes. This exercise demonstrated that dentists, with their strong background in infection control, biologic agents, collecting medical histories, and patient management, can quickly be organized into an effective, much-needed component of the catastrophe response system.

The third theme was what other additional "meaningful" training could be given in the time available. We chose to capitalize on a program developed in 2003 by the AMA in partnership with four major medical centers and three national health organizations. This training established the National Disaster Life Support (NDLS) training program to better prepare health care professionals and emergency response personnel for mass casualty events. The NDLS courses stress a comprehensive all-hazards approach to help physicians and other health professionals deal with catastrophic emergencies from terrorist acts and from explosions, fires, natural disasters (eg, hurricanes and floods), and infectious disease epidemics. The program consists of three levels of courses of increasing clinical complexity [13].

The first of this hierarchal set of training courses was chosen for its practicality and to make students aware of the possibilities for further training in the more advanced components of this program. CDLS is a 4-hour, instructor-led course designed for all public health care personnel and social workers, clergy, mental health personnel, and planners. CDLS is intended to provide a basic uniform standard of competencies, skills, and knowledge to health care and public health responders for weapons of mass destruction response. Through CDLS, the students learn the following skills:

- Define all-hazards terminology
- Recognize potential public health emergencies and their causes, risks, and consequences
- Define the D-I-S-A-S-T-E-R paradigm
- List scene priorities of a mass casualty incident response
- Describe prehospital and hospital medical components of a disaster incident response
- Describe personal protective equipment and decontamination
- Describe the role of the local public health system in public health emergencies [13].

After a didactic presentation and a short 25-question examination, the AMA offers a certificate of completion. In 2005, 320 and in 2006, 332 of NYUCD senior dental and dental hygiene students were certified on completion of the course. It was rewarding to see how "proud" our seniors were of the certificate reflecting their formal catastrophic preparedness training.

The final theme of the course addresses awareness and personal protection. NYUCD has an active emergency plan and a shelter-in-place protocol. The NYUCD student body is aware of the need for anticipating and planning for a possible attack or disaster. They are reminded that the positive behavioral response of individuals goes a long way toward mitigating the consequences of a serious event and has important implications for the practical management of a disaster scene. Using this as the basis to achieve the final course objective, the senior students were required to work in groups of four and develop either a reaction or a shelter-in-place plan for the private dental office in which they envision themselves eventually practicing. Students could tailor the plan to a specific bioterrorist agent (eg, a dirty bomb, sarin gas, a biologic weapon) or make it generic for either a natural or man-made disaster. Many students used a likely event related to the particular state in which they think they would practice. For example, earthquakes were an issue for students who planned to practice in California and tornadoes were an issue for potential mid-westerners. Faculty with a strong background in catastrophe preparedness then selected and presented to the class the most interesting and thought-provoking plans submitted and moderated the class discussions [14].

A survey was developed as a pre- and posttest to assess the attitude of the D4 students about various aspects of catastrophe preparedness. The hypothesis was that the attitudes about what were important factors about catastrophe preparedness would be changed by education. A survey was administered on the first day of the course to self-assess knowledge about bioterrorism and the students' confidence in their competency on that issue. The same survey was administered after the course was completed. Preliminary data from the study suggested that student attitudes were changed after the course. The senior students viewed more aspects of catastrophe preparedness as "important" and indicated that the educational experience made them feel more "confident" to assume a role as a responder.

Postdoctoral catastrophic preparedness training

What follows are suggestions for further training that we wanted to share with the reader. We believe that catastrophic preparedness and response training after dental school graduation has three primary targeted constituencies: (1) advanced dental training programs, (2) dentists exposed to catastrophic preparedness during their dental education who wish to learn more, and (3) dentists who have not had such training. At a minimum, all dentists should meet the proposed American Dental Education Association's proposed competencies for new graduates in practice management and informatics: "5.7. Develop a catastrophe preparedness plan for the dental practice" [3].

Advanced training programs

Dental school–based advanced training programs

Advanced dental specialty and general practice education programs based at dental schools should ensure that their postdoctoral students all have catastrophic preparedness training to the level of their dental undergraduates and any state-specific licensing continuing education requirements. Advanced dental education students should be knowledgeable of the institution's disaster plan and, for institutions that have a surge manpower response locally, be trained and integrated with that response (eg, supporting an affiliated hospital with dental students). The postdoctoral trainees should be competent in designing an office preparedness plan. Students should be made aware of advanced catastrophic training programs at the local, state, and national level (eg, the MRC) that they may wish to pursue after completion of their training. The AMA's CDLS training (4 hours) could be incorporated into the program, and successful certification could be required.

Programs that have a major hospital practice component or would expect a significant proportion of their graduates to be hospital based or affiliated should ensure that such programs consider the opportunity of introducing or reinforcing knowledge and skill sets into their medical, surgical, and anesthesia training related to catastrophic events and weapons of mass destruction. Consideration should be made for requiring completion of the AMA's BDLS training (8 hours) and additional lectures/guest speaker seminars on current topics in catastrophic response. For localities that have an MRC, advanced dental training students should be offered the opportunity to join the MRC and participate in a POD drill.

Hospital-based advanced training programs

Hospital-based advanced training programs could have additional catastrophic response training requirements because of hospitals being the focal point of receiving mass casualties. Educational objectives for hospital-based dental programs have been described in detail [8]. Five competency areas are proposed, each having several learning objectives. The learning objectives include recommended mandatory and optional knowledge and skill sets. Many of the learning objectives are already components of hospital-based training programs, including a 4-week anesthesia rotation, conducting a physical examination, and intravenous placement. Other educational objectives are easily incorporated into the residents' medical/surgical training (eg, "Describe the pathophysiology of airway burns and describe the signs and symptoms of airway burns"). These objectives reinforce much of the medical/surgical training that is already present in hospital-based curriculum. Most of the other educational objectives are met through the suggested catastrophic preparedness elements for all dental advanced training programs. Important for hospital-based training programs are the proposed educational objectives: (1) describe the hospital disaster plan, (2) complete a minimum 2-week emergency department rotation, (3) describe the military triage system, (4) describe the effects of blast and burn injuries, (5) describe the principles and practice of a mass decontamination station, (6) describe the use of personal protective barriers for biologic agents and how they differ from standard universal precautions, and (7) describe the setup and practice of a POD system. An opportunity for the trainees to be certified in the AMA's ADLS course (16 hours) should be considered. Attending dentists who are affiliated with the hospital-based training programs also should meet the proposed competencies and acquire the corresponding knowledge and skill sets.

The catastrophic preparedness and response training delineated for the dental advanced training programs will establish a cadre of knowledgeable and skilled dental practitioners who are an asset to their communities and provide leadership in the dental profession and, for some, will be an entry point to greater involvement with disaster response programs and systems.

Continuing education for the practicing dentist

In the near future, the members of the practicing dental profession will consist of these two sets of dentists: dentists educated and trained in their pre- and postdoctoral years in catastrophic preparedness and response and dentists who graduated before the development and implementation of the educational objectives. Continuing education on catastrophic preparedness and response will have two audiences for a period of time, with a potential third group of dentists who wish to be formal members of disaster response official organizations.

It should be expected that practicing dentists who do not graduate with catastrophic preparedness and response training will have courses available to allow them to meet the competencies for the dental schools and those currently proposed for new graduates. All practicing dentists should have an opportunity to learn the elements of developing an office preparedness plan. Emerging catastrophic preparedness issues should be addressed in continuing education (eg, avian flu: the science and response planning). A knowledge of catastrophic event response plans/organizations and opportunities for dentists should be provided by all state dental societies. Derived from these plans/organizations and opportunities for dentists' information, continuing educational pathways should be provided that allow practicing dentists to develop additional competencies. The AMA's disaster life support courses are an example of this. Information regarding sources of online self-education and training (eg, www.chip.med.nyu.edu) should be made readily available to busy practitioners.

Graduates who have had catastrophic preparedness and response competencies addressed in pre- and postdoctoral training will have a continuing educational need for periodic updating of their knowledge and skills. These dentists also will be initially more "attuned" to the subject and may have a greater preference in many cases for pathways through continuing education for more advanced topics/training. It can be expected that these practitioners will be able to provide local and district dental societies with knowledge and expertise for planning and developing key continuing education programs. They will assume leadership roles at local and district level in coordinating real involvement opportunities for dentists in catastrophic response plans.

A subset of the dental profession will become more officially part of catastrophic response organizations. Several programs are available to these interested dentists, including the Department of Homeland Security Citizen Corps program, which administers the Community Emergency Response Team (CERT) and MRC programs and is responsible for the national disaster medical systems, which contains several subprograms [15]. CERT is a citizen volunteer program based at the local level that trains civilians as auxiliary responders to disasters and prepares volunteers for more routine daily emergencies. The MRC is a system to incorporate trained and credentialed health and public health personnel to be available to respond to mass disasters (ie, a surge demand manpower resource). This organization functions at local, regional, and national levels but is primarily organized at the local level to meet a particular community's specific needs.

For dentists who wish to be part of a national level disaster response, the National Disaster Medical System (NDMS) is available. This system is a federal organization of multiple units capable of supporting local and state level response to disasters. There are several types of NDMS units, each type composed of multiple regional based teams. Historically, dentists have been key members of the Disaster Mortuary Operational Response Teams; however, well-trained and interested dental professionals may have the opportunity to serve with a Disaster Medical Assistance Team (DMAT). Personnel of DMATs include medical and paraprofessional medical personnel. After catastrophic events, disaster medical assistance team duties include triaging patients, providing emergency medical care, and preparing for the evacuation of patients. The units also can provide primary health care if the local health systems are unable to meet demand after a disaster [16].

References

[1] Guay AH. Dentistry's response to bioterrorism: a report of a consensus workshop. J Am Dent Assoc 2002;133:1181–7.

[2] Chmar JE, Ranney RR, Guay AH, et al. Incorporating bioterrorism training into dental education: report of ADA-ADEA terrorism and mass casualty curriculum development workshop. J Dent Educ 2004;68:1196–9.

[3] Association of Dental Schools (ADEA) House of Delegates. Competencies for the new general dentist. Available at: http://www.adea.org/cci/CallforComments09292006.pdf. Accessed December 10, 2006.

[4] Psoter W, Glotzer DL. A summary report on the expansion of the role of dentists and their enhancement of the medical surge response. New York: NYU College of Dentistry; 2005. Available from: http://www.chip.med.nyu.edu. Accessed December 10, 2006.

[5] Steigbigel NH, Blaser MJ, Brewer K, et al. Enhancing medical and public health capabilities during times of crisis: a grant from the Department of Justice, Office of Justice Programs. 202-DT-CX-K002, New York; 2005.
[6] Janousek JT, De Lorenzo RA, Coppola M. Mass casualty triage knowledge of military medical personnel. Mil Med 1999;164:332–5.
[7] AMA. National disaster life support. 2003; Available at: http://www.ama-assn.org/ama/pub/category/12606.html. Accessed June 8, 2005.
[8] Glotzer D, Rinchiuso A, Rekow D, et al. The medical reserve corps: an opportunity for dentists to serve. N Y State Dent J 2006;72(1):60–1.
[9] Clinical Triage course, SoM., Department of Emergency Medicine. Triage: recognizing clinical syndromes for disasters. Basic recognition of clinical syndromes associated with biological, chemical and radioactive agents. Available at: http://chip.med.nyu.edu/course/view.php?id=36. Accessed December 10, 2006.
[10] More FG, Phelan J, Boylan R, et al. Predoctoral dental school curriculum for catastrophe preparedness. J Dent Educ 2004;68:851–8.
[11] Glotzer DL, More FG, Phelan J, et al. Introducing a senior course on catastrophe preparedness into the dental school curriculum. J Dent Educ 2006;70:225–30.
[12] Medical Reserve Corps, Office of Surgeon General. Available at: http://www.medicalreservecorps.gov. Accessed January 10, 2006.
[13] AMA (CPHPDR). Core disaster life support (CDLS). Available at: http://www.ama-assn.org/ama/pub/category/12607.html. Accessed July 25, 2005.
[14] Glotzer DL, More FG. Compilation of senior dental student submissions on protective action plans submitted as course requirement. Results available upon request.
[15] Briggs SM, Brinsfield KH. Advanced disaster medical response: manual for providers. Boston (MA): Harvard Medical International Trauma & Disaster Institute; 2003.
[16] Programs, Preparedness & Response. Department of Homeland Security. Available at: http://www.dhs.gov/xprepresp/programs/. Accessed November 15, 2005.

ELSEVIER
SAUNDERS

THE DENTAL CLINICS OF NORTH AMERICA

Dent Clin N Am 51 (2007) 819–825

National Disaster Life Support Programs: A Platform for Multi-Disciplinary Disaster Response

Phillip L. Coule, MD, FACEP[a,*], Jack A. Horner, BS[a,b]

[a]*Department of Emergency Medicine, Center of Operational Medicine, Medical College of Georgia, AF2036, 1120 15th Street, Augusta, GA 30912, USA*
[b]*National Disaster Life Support Foundation, Inc., USA*

Human nature is inclined to respond to disasters by whatever means available, and dental professionals are no different. Historically, hundreds of volunteers have turned out to assist in response to floods, earthquakes, hurricanes, explosions, and disasters of every conceivable type. The motivation is generally one of compassion for our fellow humans and a sincere desire to help. In recent years it has been recognized that response of untrained volunteers can be counterproductive and can lead to serious risks to the multitude of responders. The role of dental health professionals during a disaster has historically been ill defined. The role of dental health professionals in identifying remains of victims is well documented in diverse multiple incidents from plane crashes to mass graves [1–3]. A training program in Australia focuses on better preparing dental professionals to perform dental autopsy for this vital function [4].

Displaced persons from natural disasters need emergency and routine dental care. Relegating dental professionals to these two roles only during disasters would be short sighted, imprudent, and illogical. Dental professionals are, first and foremost, health care providers with knowledge of anatomy, physiology, medication administration, and emergency interventions. With proper training, dental providers can become a force multiplier for other emergency responders to disasters of various types. Some states already have enacted laws that expand the dental provider's scope of practice during a disaster [5].

The importance of proper training cannot be understated. We must recognize that the first responders to a disaster scene, despite their noble intent,

* Corresponding author.
E-mail address: pcoule@mcg.edu (P.L. Coule).

doi:10.1016/j.cden.2007.06.006 ***dental.theclinics.com***

are unaware of the precise cause of the event and, more importantly, are unaware of the possible secondary consequences of the event. It may be apparent that an explosion has occurred, but was it accidental or intentional? Did it result in the dispersion of dangerous chemicals into the scene? Are biologic or radioactive agents contaminating the area? Is there a likelihood of secondary explosions that could jeopardize the responders' safety? Are there structural or environmental threats as a result of the event? These are among the many reasons why dental professionals and all first responders should approach a disaster scene with a careful and systematic approach—an all-hazards approach. The alternative risk is that they may become secondary victims of the event, thereby increasing the number of victims and reducing the number of effective responders. Proper training must prepare responders to consider various hazards and means by which to mitigate their effects. This article describes one such training program (the National Disaster Life Support [NDLS] program) as a possible means to prepare dental providers to better respond to disasters and describes a simple triage technique that can be used by dental professionals to triage patients.

A commonality of approach to disasters is vital to an effective response [6]. A community can have the best trained fire personnel, the most competent and well-trained paramedics, and the best trained police imaginable, but if they are not trained in a manner that facilitates working cohesively, their disparate training can result in less-than-optimal effectiveness—it can be counterproductive.

Recognizing the need for a common approach, a group of personnel from four academic institutions—the Medical College of Georgia, the University of Georgia, the University of Texas Southwestern Medical Center, and the University of Texas School of Public Health–Houston—partnered in an effort to develop a standardized all-hazards curriculum for the training of responder personnel. Congressional funding was sought for support of the developmental effort, and Senator Max Cleland (D-GA) proposed the initiative on the floor of the US Senate on September 10, 2001 [7]. The events of the next day underscored the importance of the proposed effort. Funding was made available through the Centers for Disease Control and Prevention, and subsequently a partnership with the American Medical Association and American College of Emergency Physicians was formed.

The result was a family of courses, called the NDLS courses, to provide awareness level to operations level training to a multidisciplinary spectrum of providers from first responders to advanced in-hospital care. These courses, Core Disaster Life Support (CDLS), Basic Disaster Life Support (BDLS), Advanced Disaster Life Support (ADLS), and NDLS decontamination, are designed to create interoperable providers across the spectrum of personnel, and dental professionals are no exception.

The CDLS course is a 4-hour awareness level course directed at nonmedical personnel. The course lays the foundation on which the entire family of NDLS courses is based. This foundation consists of several unique memory mnemonics that serve to facilitate recall of key response components otherwise easily overlooked under the stress of emergency response.

The BDLS course is the introductory course for medical personnel, including emergency medical technicians, paramedics, nurses, physicians, dentists, veterinarians, and other health care providers. The content is based on the DISASTER paradigm for each of the topics, including triage, natural disasters, traumatic and explosive events, chemical events, biologic events, nuclear/radiation events, and psychological consequences. Additional topics provide a well-rounded opportunity for understanding the complex aspects of disaster consequences.

The ADLS course is a 2-day practical, hands-on, training program that covers the practical aspects of rendering aid to the unique kinds of injuries to be found at a disaster scene. The topics covered include patient treatment procedures, mass prophylaxis, patient decontamination, mass triage, and associated skills.

The fourth course is NDLS-decontamination. This course provides operational level training in the procedures of patient decontamination. It addresses the fact that typically to reserve medical personnel for care delivery, a hospital staffs a decontamination team with nonmedical individuals. This team can include personnel from public safety, maintenance, and housekeeping. It is imperative that these teams understand the policies and procedures of decontamination and have an opportunity to actually conduct practice on mock victims.

All of the NDLS courses are organized around a unifying mnemonic called the DISASTER paradigm:

D: Detect
I: Incident command
S: Safety and security
A: Assess hazards
S: Support
T: Triage and treatment
E: Evacuation
R: Recovery

Each topic addressed in each course is structured around this unifying theme.

One of the most vital functions that a dental health provider can provide during a disaster is triage, or the sorting of victims into priorities of treatment. Controversy exists over the manner and method of the triage of disaster victims. The NDLS courses teach a simple type of triage called MASS triage:

M: Move
A: Assess
S: Sort
S: Send

MASS triage is based on the fact that the gross motor component of the Glasgow Coma Scale and systolic blood pressure is a good predictor of mortality from trauma [8,9]. **"Id-me"** Is an easy-to-remember phrase that incorporates a mnemonic device for sorting patients during mass casualty incident (MCI) triage into **I**mmediate, **D**elayed, **M**inimal, and **E**xpectant.

Mass triage "MOVE"

The initial challenge in triage is to determine accurately which patients need immediate lifesaving care versus which patients are simply demanding immediate attention. Victims screaming and calling for help, scene confusion, victims wandering around the area, and a multitude of other distractions can limit your effectiveness. The first step in triaging a large group of patients is to ask them to move. For example, if a large group of patients is congregated, one might shout, "Everyone who can hear me and needs medical attention, please move to the area with the green flag." Believing that they will receive medical care more quickly, the ambulatory patients likely will move to the designated area. Patients who are able to ambulate should, by virtue of this fact, have an intact airway, breathing, circulation, and blood pressure adequate enough to sustain an ambulatory position. This group of patients who is able to ambulate to another location should be considered "minimal" for a triage group category during this initial triage step. Because this initial step groups patients without individual assessment of each patient, some individuals may have conditions that worsen and result in a more urgent triage category.

The second step of the "MOVE" of MASS triage is to ask the remaining victims to move an arm or leg. For example, say to the remaining victims, "Everyone who can hear me, please raise an arm or leg so we can come help you." To follow this command, the victim must have sufficient vital signs for them to remain conscious, hear the instructions, and follow commands but be unable to ambulate because of injury or other serious conditions. This patient group is considered the initial delayed group for a triage category (Fig. 1).

The third step of the "MOVE" of MASS triage is to identify immediately the patients who could not complete the first two steps. Patients who are not moving at all are the first priority for assessment. Expectant and dead patients are also among this group.

Mass triage "ASSESS"

After the steps outlined in "MOVE" are completed, it is time to "ASSESS." "MOVE" should group patients into **I**mmediate, **D**elayed, and **M**inimal initial groups to order the initial sorting of individual patient assessments more effectively. The initial focus for the immediate group is

"MOVE" of MASS Triage		
Goal:	**Action:**	**"ID-me" Category:**
Group ambulatory patients	"Everyone who can hear me and needs medical attention, please move to the area with the green flag".	Minimal initial group
Group awake, follow commands	Ask the remaining victims "everyone who can hear me please raise an arm or leg so we can come help you"	Delayed initial group
Identify who is left	Proceed immediately to these patients and deliver immediate life-saving interventions.	Immediate initial group

Fig. 1. Move of MASS triage.

airway, breathing, circulation, and performing life saving interventions such as stopping exsanguinating hemorrhage. The health care provider should assess for unresponsiveness. For patients who are unresponsive, the airway should be opened and the breathing assessed. Patients who are not breathing are considered expectant. Patients who are breathing but unresponsive are immediate or expectant, depending on the severity of injury. If a quick initial survey of the victim reveals wounds that are likely to be fatal, the patient is considered expectant.

Mass triage "SORT"

After "ASSESS" and the immediate life-threatening interventions have been completed, the next step is to "SORT" the patients into one of four triage categories. **"Id-me"** is an easy-to-remember phrase that incorporates a mnemonic for sorting patients during MCI triage into **I**mmediate, **D**elayed, **M**inimal, and **E**xpectant groups.

Immediate patients have an obvious threat to life or limb.

Delayed patients who are in need of definitive medical care but should not decompensate rapidly if the care is delayed initially.

Minimal patients are the "walking wounded."

Expectant patients have little or no chance of survival despite maximum therapy; therefore, resources are not used initially to care for them unless resources become available.

Mass triage "SEND"

After the "SORT" is operational and while treatment is ongoing, it is important to focus on "SEND," or transporting patients away from the scene.

The disposition options for patients are to be treated and released from the scene or sent to hospitals, secondary treatment facilities, or morgue facilities based on their triage category and clinical status.

In summary of triage, the use of the MASS triage model simplifies the process of triaging large numbers of patients while maintaining a simple, common terminology that allows for improved coordination between civilian and military assets responding to an MCI. Dental professionals can perform mass triage and bring some order to a triage scene.

Shortly after the events of September 11, the American Medical Association established the Center for Disaster Preparedness and Emergency Response. This center partnered with the NDLS program to further the dissemination of this standardized all-hazards training. To date, more than 50,000 individuals have received NDLS training, with courses conducted in more than 40 states. NDLS courses also have been conducted in eight foreign countries, with dental professionals being among the individuals trained. In 2004, the Academic Partners, together with the American Medical Association, established a nonprofit foundation, the National Disaster Life Support Foundation. One of the primary purposes of the foundation is to oversee the establishment of affiliated training centers for the conduct of the courses. Currently, there are almost 50 such accredited centers representing 20 states.

The motivation to develop the NDLS courses was to standardize the all-hazards training and build a framework around which separate groups responding to the same disaster could function collaboratively. It should not matter that teams or pools of personnel are from different parts of the country—the NDLS courses provide them with the wherewithal to function as "one team." Such training can mean the difference between chaos and concert at the scene of the event. A cadre of 50 students attending an ADLS course might easily represent a mix of emergency medical technicians, paramedics, nurses, dentists, emergency managers, surgeons, family practice physicians, and other medical specialties. During a typical MASS casualty exercise, it is reassuring to observe such diverse backgrounds working cohesively as a team as they assess the condition of a high-fidelity computerized patient simulator presenting symptoms of injury and make decisions regarding appropriate care. It is equally rewarding to observe the same team's approach to the scene of a mass casualty event and exercise the appropriate cautions regarding safety and security. It has become abundantly clear that the incorporation of standardized training across all disciplines has provided a mechanism for effective multidisciplinary integration.

References

[1] Petju M, Suteerayongprasert A, Thongpud R, et al. Importance of dental records for victim identification following the Indian Ocean tsunami disaster in Thailand. Public Health 2007;251–7.

[2] Roman Bux, Heidemann Detlef, Enders Markus, et al. The value of examination aids in victim identification: a retrospective study of an airplane crash in Nepal in 2002. Forensic Sci Int 2006;164(2–3):155–8.
[3] Taylor PT, Wilson ME, Lyons TJ. Forensic odontology lessons: multi-shooting incident at Port Arthur, Tasmania. Forensic Sci Int 2002;130(2–3):174–82.
[4] Griffiths CJ, Parker D, Middleton A. Forensic dental training in Australia. Forensic Sci Int 1988;36(3–4):279–82.
[5] Colvard MD, Lampiris LN, Cordell GA, et al. The dental emergency responder: expanding the scope of dental practice. J Am Dent Assn 2006;137(4):68–73.
[6] Coule PL, Dallas C, Schwartz RB, et al, editors. Basic disaster life support version 2.5. Chicago: American Medical Association; 2003.
[7] Congressional Record. Hon Senator Max Cleland. Sept 10, 2001. p. S9245.
[8] Meredith W, Rutledge R, Hanson AR, et al. Field triage of trauma patients based on the ability to follow commands: a study in 29,573 patients. J Trauma 1995;38(1):129–35.
[9] Garner A, Lee A, Harrison K, et al. Comparative analysis of multiple-casualty incident triage algorithms. Ann Emerg Med 2001;38(5):541–8.

ELSEVIER
SAUNDERS

Dent Clin N Am 51 (2007) 827–835

THE DENTAL CLINICS OF NORTH AMERICA

TOPOFF 2 and the Inclusion of Dental Professionals into Federal Exercise Design and Execution

James C. Hagen, PhD, MBA, MPH, CERC, MEP[a,*], Beverly Parota, RDH, MEd, MBA, CERC[a,b], Mila Tsagalis, RDH, MPH[b]

[a]*Graham School of Management, Saint Xavier University, 3700 West 103rd Street, Chicago, IL 60655, USA*
[b]*DuPage County Health Department, 111 N. County Farm Road, Wheaton, IL 60187, USA*

The vulnerability of our nation to disasters, both natural and man-made, has become abundantly clear in recent years. It is necessary that we use the composite knowledge, creativity, expertise, and all available human resources if we hope to successfully prepare for, respond to, and recover from these devastating events. Our concept of man-made disasters has been tragically broadened from accidental chemical spills and nuclear reactor radiation leaks to the horror of terrorism in all of its destructive forms. We have become familiar with such terms as asymmetrical warfare, the unthinkable tactics used when another belief system or country fights someone much stronger or of greater military might. We are haunted by the visions of death and disease as we consider and create scenarios for pandemic influenza.

In the past, the dental professional's role in disasters has been limited to the field of forensic dentistry [1–4]. In real life, through forensic dentistry and the application of dental and paradental knowledge, the living and the dead can be identified. In some cases, cause of death can be determined, with all of the associated legal and criminal ramifications. In the unreal world of theater and film, however, the dental profession is often portrayed somewhat differently. Films have evoked images of dentists as villains and evil indeed. The former Nazi torturer, Dr. Christian Szell (Lawrence Olivier), used his dental drill to torture Thomas Levy (Dustin Hoffman) in the

* Corresponding author.
E-mail address: hagen@sxu.edu (J.C. Hagen).

doi:10.1016/j.cden.2007.07.001
dental.theclinics.com

1976 film "Marathon Man." Then there were the insane dentists: Dr. Alan Feinstone (Corbin Bernsen) as the murdering dentist from the 1996 movie "Dentist" and Dr. Orin Scrivello (Steve Martin) in the 1986 cult classic "Little Shop of Horrors."

Far beyond these images, both real and imagined, lies the much greater perspective of the role and importance of the trained dental professional during times of crisis [5–10]. The role of the dental professional as a source of information, reassurance, medical care, dispensing of antimicrobial agents or vaccines, and guidance during a disaster must not be minimized. If we are to survive as a nation after disaster, we must use all of the resources, training, and expertise at our disposal. This article examines the dental professional's role in emergency management activities, specifically related to design and execution of such federal exercises as the Top Officials (TOPOFF) series. Experiences from the Chicago TOPOFF 2 exercise are used as an example.

The effects that a massive disaster can have on society and resulting societal disruption have been seen clearly here and abroad in recent years. Hurricane Katrina was a defining moment for us in preparedness and response to natural disaster, as was the 2004 Indian Ocean tsunami on a global scale and September 11th for homeland security in the United States. The stark realization of our vulnerability and desperate need for preparedness and interaction of sectors became abundantly clear. Historically, dental professionals, including dentists, hygienists, dental assistants, laboratory technicians, and all others considered to be dental auxiliaries, have been poorly used in these national response activities [5,6]. This lack of involvement has resulted in a plethora of questions as to their importance should an event actually occur.

Potential roles for the dental professional

There are many areas in which dental professionals may provide assistance, depending on the specifics of the disaster and needs of the community [8,11–13]. The following list includes a few of those areas, as suggested by Dr. Guay and others:

- Surveillance and notification
- Diagnosis and monitoring
- Referral
- Medications
- Triage
- Medical care augmentation
- Decontamination and infection control

The vital need for persons to assist with medical tasks takes on new meaning when considering that only 50% of health care workers (eg, doctors, nurses, and hospital workers) said they would report to work during a potential outbreak of avian flu [14]. Experts suggest that a specific dental emergency response plan, along with its own command and control structure, be in place [15]. This plan must be fully integrated into the overall area plan and well communicated to the professional dental societies.

Alfano stated that "One group that will be ready, based on the ADA's leadership, is the nation's dentists, who will play a far more important role in preparedness and response than anyone ever imagined in the dark days of September 2001" [16]. A central role for public health in disasters involving infectious diseases, and one in which nontraditional professionals could be of great importance, would be at the points of dispensing (PODs) of antibiotics and vaccines. This area is of vital importance to decreasing disease-associated morbidity and mortality. In many cases, the needed tasks are part of the day-to-day routines for individuals in the dental profession.

1. As people entered the POD, visual triage would take place to identify and remove persons who are exhibiting symptoms. In the dental office, patients would be viewed in a holistic manner. Skin, eyes, gum tissue, voice, and stature would be appraised while seating the patient.
2. Individuals seeking medications at the POD would be required to complete a medication administration record or a mini health history. These documents would be reviewed before movement into the dispensing area. Questions would be asked regarding medications or illnesses that could preclude them from receiving certain medications. Every patient in a dental office is requested to complete a medical history form regularly and update at each visit. The members of the dental team would review these documents and provide services accordingly.
3. Regardless of the type of medications dispensed at the PODs, whether injections or pills, dentists and hygienists are trained to provide them. These skills are required when attempting to prevent the spread of a pandemic or other type of disease. States may have certain restrictions, but based on emergency powers acts, these restrictions may be lifted in a major public health event. In dental practices across the country, dentists give injections daily. Some states give this same licensure to hygienists.
4. Use of personal protective equipment may be necessary. First responders and individuals called upon to assist must know how to use and remove personal protective equipment. The members of the dental team have long used masks, gloves, smocks, and aprons. Their expertise could be taught to persons who are called upon to assist during an emergency of this type.
5. Certain areas of the POD would have to be cleaned to ensure an aseptic field. This is an area of expertise held by workers in the dental field and a skill needed at the PODs.
6. Dental professionals are trained in cardiopulmonary resuscitation and first aid, skills that are greatly needed during disasters of any type.

7. Dentists have expansive knowledge and great credibility. They are recognized leaders and members of social and philanthropic groups. They are well known for "giving back" to their neighborhoods and could recruit other volunteers to assist in the emergency operations.
8. Dental professionals have knowledge of the many community resources. Many have provided services in schools and are aware of how best to care for children.
9. Dental professionals are excellent at record keeping, another critical skill needed for the recovery phase.
10. Dentists and hygienists could be recruited easily through their professional societies. The requirement for continuing education credit would make the education desirable.

Evolution of the federal Top Officials series of exercises

Before the September 11th attack and in response to such events as the 1995 sarin gas attack in the Tokyo subway, in 1988, Congress mandated that the Department of State and Department of Defense conduct a series of challenging role-playing exercises that involved federal, state, and local levels [17]. They would be national level, multiagency, multi-jurisdictional, real-time, limited notice events in response to terrorism involving weapons of mass destruction. The TOPOFF events are held in various locations in the United States and abroad.

TOPOFF 1, 2000: Portsmouth, New Hampshire and Denver, Colorado
TOPOFF 2, 2003: Chicago area, Illinois, Seattle area, Washington, and Canada
TOPOFF 3, 2005: Union and Middlesex counties in New Jersey, New London, Connecticut, and the United Kingdom
TOPOFF 4, 2007: Portland, Oregon, Phoenix, Arizona, and Guam (to be held in October 2007)

Homeland Security exercise and evaluation program

The Homeland Security exercise and evaluation program (HSEEP) was designed to assist state and local governments in developing and implementing a state exercise and evaluation program to assess and enhance domestic preparedness [18]. Homeland Security Directive Number 8 [19] directed that the Department of Homeland Security, in coordination with other appropriate federal departments and agencies, establish a "national program and a multi-year planning system to conduct homeland security preparedness-related exercises that reinforces identified training standards, provides for evaluation of readiness, and supports the National Preparedness Goal." HSEEP provides the program structure, multiyear planning system, tools, and guidance necessary to build and sustain exercise programs that enhance homeland security capabilities and preparedness [20]. HSEEP is described as a capabilities and performance-based exercise program that provides a standardized policy, methodology, and language for designing, developing, conducting, and evaluating all exercises. All HSEEP exercise design objectives draw from the target capabilities list. Fifteen national scenarios were created as the worst case scenarios for natural and man-made disasters [21,22]. The target capabilities list was created from a consideration of all the capabilities needed to respond to these disasters. The Department of Homeland Security has released its latest draft of the target capabilities list, in which specific areas of activity for dental professionals can be found [23].

All HSEEP material can be found on the Department of Homeland Security Web site, including the five instructional volumes of the program [20].

Volume 1: HSEEP overview and exercise program management
Volume 2: Exercise planning and conduct
Volume 3: Exercise evaluation and improvement planning
Volume 4: Sample exercise documents, formats, multimedia files, and policy guidance for exercise planning
Volume 5: Prevention exercises

Volumes 1 to 3 are new editions for 2007, whereas Volume 5 is currently in draft form and undergoing revisions. The site contains a wealth of information for individuals involved in exercise design and execution.

Top Officials 2

As terrorist events escalated in the world and the September 11th attack rocked our country, the TOPOFF event took on new significance, and plans to involve all sectors were translated into action. TOPOFF 2 was held in 2003 in Chicago, Illinois, Seattle, Washington, and Canada [24]. T2 was the most comprehensive and the largest terrorism response exercise to have been conducted in the United States. From May 12 to May 16, an exercise scenario was played out in which a terrorist organization detonated a radiologic dispersal device in Seattle, Washington as a diversion for the real attack, which was a covert release of pneumonic plague at three metropolitan Chicago locations. These locations included Union Station, the United Center during a Blackhawk's game, and the international terminal at O'Hare International Airport. The complex exercise also included significant pre-exercise intelligence play, a cyber attack, and credible threats against other locations. The exercise brought together 25 federal, state, and local agencies to test and examine domestic incident response. Although this was labeled as a TOPOFF event, individuals at the local level were most deeply involved in the full-scale exercise. It was realized that this was as an opportunity to test our systems and ability to respond to the horrific scenario.

DuPage County, Illinois was one of the local venues for full-scale play in the TOPOFF 2 exercise. Our experience was at a county government level, through which all local resources and coordination occurred [25], including the medical and medical surge response and coordination of the distribution and dispensing of medications to first responders and the general public. Integral in the response was one of the incident commanders (a former professor and assistant dean for research at Chicago's Loyola School of Dentistry), the certified emergency response coordinator and primary author of the response plan (a Registered Dental Hygenist [RDH] and former dental health program manager), and the current program manager for dental health services (also an RDH). The other public health dental hygienists and dental staff were assigned specific roles in the event. These participants were in positions to clearly observe the sequence of events and determine the successes and challenges of the public health and medical systems in response to a simulated release of pneumonic plague. At that time in DuPage County, a medical reserve corps had just been initiated. There were approximately 900 volunteers, including approximately 40 dental health professionals such as dentists, hygienists, and dental auxiliaries.

Psoter and Glotzer's report to Department of Justice [26] stated that the use of nontraditional medical and public health professionals in a surge environment would depend on how committed the leaderships of the medical and dental professions were to the concept and envisioned roles. Before—and at the time of—the TOPOFF 2 event, officers of the West Suburban Branch of the Chicago Dental Society and the West Suburban Dental Hygienists Association were approached, and they agreed that during an emergency, society members would respond to assigned locations and assume roles as dispensers of antibiotics or assist the community in any way necessary.

The incident commander coordinated all public health activities, including performing the epidemiologic investigation, assisting in all manners of public information and communication, and distributing and dispensing antimicrobials through our PODs. The emergency response coordinator was responsible for creating the emergency operations procedures, operations section plan, and strategic national stockpile annex and developing the all hazards plan. She acted as one of the strategic national stockpile coordinators, sat in the command center as operations chief and part of command staff, briefed the county crisis management team, and assisted in the development of press messages. The dental health services program manager acted as a triage manager, conducting triage at the POD and assisting in the coordination of the strategic national stockpile site. Dental hygienists assisted in the clinic area by working as health educators and registration and inventory clerks. Dental clerks and assistants registered, interpreted, assisted in completion of documentation, and were inventory clerks who distributed medications to the dispensers.

One fact that became clear as TOPOFF 2 unfolded was that even within the public health realm, the need for medically trained staff far exceeded the number of persons who would be needed to staff and maintain the dispensing sites for antibiotics or vaccines. There was also a need for individuals trained as managers to be able to direct the PODs. When added to the after-action reports from all three TOPOFF events, this need would have to be added to the drastic shortage of medical personnel in the health care system. The worst case scenario of overwhelming shortage is only now being envisioned in the plans and exercises being developed for potential pandemic influenza in our nation.

Changing legislation and defined training requirements

The environment for potential inclusion of nontraditional assistance is changing through legislation and defined training requirements (even during initial training). The dental profession's organized leadership sees a role, if not an obligation, for dental professionals to help meet surge needs for additional medical assistance. Discussions are beginning concerning specific training to be required. Galligan [27] highlighted the need for California dental health care workers to obtain additional training to augment existing medical professionals during a declared emergency. From survey data of oral health care professionals who have taken the American Medical Association's national disaster life support training curriculum, Colvard and colleagues [28] concluded that the core disaster life support and basic disaster life support training were of "great educational value."

Of vital importance have been two pieces of legislation that will allow a wider scope of practice for dental professionals during a declared disaster [5]. Public Act 94-409, effective January 1, 2006, defines the dental emergency responder within the Dental Practice Act. A dental emergency responder is a dentist or dental hygienist certified by the State of Illinois in Emergency Medicine who is acting within the scope of practice when administering total body care during a declared local, state, or federal emergency as part of a recognized response organization. Through National Disaster Life Support-level certification courses, Illinois Medical Emergency Response Team (IMERT) training, and certification, oral health care professionals can become registered within the IMERT response database as dental emergency responders.

Another legislative action of great importance is Public Act 94-733, which allows the Secretary of the Illinois Department of Financial and Professional Regulation to expand the scope of practice of professionals licensed in Illinois if under the direction of the Illinois Department of Public Health and the Illinois Emergency Management Agency. These pieces of legislation will potentially open the doors for more effective use of the expertise of dental professionals during disasters. Great strides are being made in proposing educational objectives [26] and incorporating a senior course on catastrophic preparedness into dental school curricula [29].

Summary

The impact of current thought, legislation, and collaborations has not been felt within the TOPOFF construct. It is hoped that as TOPOFF 4 is designed for fall of 2008, the ability to expand and enhance our capacity to respond through cooperation and coordination of all health care professionals can be tested. Dental professionals must take this on as an obligation and responsibility. Methods for better preparation for disasters is available through continuing education or through programs provided by state public health departments and emergency management agencies will make this possible. It is also encouraged that exercise, both discussion-based and operations-based will be designed and executed that specifically test these areas of preparedness and response. It is through use of certified Master Exercise Planners, the HSEEP process, and appropriate designation of Task Capabilities and objectives that we can better prepare for the challenges ahead.

References

[1] DeValck E. Major incident response: collecting ante-mortem data. Forensic Sci Int 2006; 159(Suppl 1):S15–9.
[2] Bajaj A. Disaster victim identification: tsunami. Br Dent J 2005;198:504–5.
[3] Clark DH. An analysis of forensic odontology in ten mass disasters. Int Dent J 1994;44(3): 241–50.
[4] Pretty IA, Webb DA, Sweet D. The design and assessment of mock disasters for dental personnel. J Forensic Sci 2001;46(1):74–9.
[5] Colvard MD, Lampiris LN, Cordell GA, et al. The dental emergency responder: expanding the scope of dental practice. J Am Dent Assoc 2006;137(4):468–73.
[6] Hobson K. Are we ready? Available at: http://health.usnews.com/usnews/health/articles/060501/1disaster.htm. Accessed June 29, 2007.
[7] NY State Dental Foundation. Guiding principles underlying NYSDA policies with respect to planning for catastrophic events and public health threats. Available at: http://www.nysdental.org/emergency_response/emergency_plan.cfm. Accessed June 27, 2007.
[8] Guay A. Dentistry's response to bioterrorism: a report of a consensus workshop. J Am Dent Assoc 2002;133(9):1181–7.
[9] Psoter WJ, Triola MM, Morse DE, et al. Enhancing medical and public health capabilities during times of crisis: a summary report on the expansion of the role of dentists and their enhancement of the medical surge response. N Y State Dent J 2003;69:25–7.
[10] Morlag WM. Dentistry's vital role in disaster preparedness. J Calif Dent Assoc 1996;24(5): 63–6.
[11] ADA Conference Summary. Dentistry's role in responding to bioterrorism and other catastrophic events. Available at: http://www.ada.org/prof/resources/topics/topics_bioterrorism_conf.pdf. Accessed March 27–28, 2003.
[12] Guay AH. Dentistry's vital role in disaster preparedness. J Calif Dent Assoc 1996;24(5): 63–6.
[13] Downes EJ. We've got the skills: let's use them. N Y State Dent J 2003;69(5):24.

[14] Medical News Today. Will the healthcare workers go to work during disasters? Available at: www.medicalnewstoday.com/printerfriendlynews.php?newsid=70828. Accessed June 29, 2007.
[15] American Dental Association. Dentistry's response to bioterrorism and other mass disasters: a template for dental societies to use in developing a plan for providing assistance in the response to a bioterrorism attack and other mass disasters. Available at: http://www.ada.org/prof/resources/topics/topics_bioterrorism.pdf. Accessed June 29, 2007.
[16] Alfano MC. Bioterrorism response. J Am Dent Assoc 2003;134(3):2T76.
[17] Department of State. TOPOFF (Top Officials). Available at: http://www.state.gov/s/ct/rls/fs/2002/12129.htm. Accessed June 29, 2007.
[18] Department of Homeland Security. Welcome to the HSEEP website. Available at: https://hseep.dhs.gov/default.htm. Accessed June 30, 2007.
[19] The White House. December 17, 2003 Homeland Security Presidential Directive/Hspd-8. Available at: http://www.whitehouse.gov/news/releases/2003/12/20031217-6.html. Accessed August 14, 2007.
[20] Department of Homeland Security. About HSEEP: frequently asked questions. Available at: https://hseep.dhs.gov/faq.htm#q10. Accessed June 29, 2007.
[21] Homeland Security Council. National planning scenarios: executive summaries. Available at: http://cees.tamiu.edu/covertheborder/TOOLS/NationalPlanningSen.pdf. Accessed June 23, 2007.
[22] Brookings Institute. Planning scenarios and summary descriptions. Available at: http://www.brookings.edu/views/testimony/ohanlon/20051026_3.pdf. Accessed June 29, 2007.
[23] Department of Homeland Security. Lessons learned information sharing. Available at: http://www.llis.gov. Accessed June 30, 2007.
[24] Department of Homeland Security. Top officials (TOPOFF) exercise series: TOPOFF 2. After action summary report for public release. Available at: http://biotech.law.lsu.edu/blaw/dhs/TOPOFF2_Report_Final_Public.PDF. Accessed June 23, 2007.
[25] Hagen JC. Local public health department as surveillance gatekeeper. In: O'Leary M, editor. The first 72 hours: a community approach to disaster preparedness. New York: iUniverse, Inc.; 2004. p. 293–304.
[26] Psoter WJ, Herman NG, More FG, et al. Proposed educational objectives for hospital-based dentists during catastrophic events and disaster response. J Dent Educ 2006;70(8):835–43.
[27] Galligan JM. Dentists can contribute expertise in a major public health disaster. J Calif Dent Assoc 2004;32(8):701–8.
[28] Colvard MD, Naiman MI, Mata D, et al. Disaster medicine training survey results for dental health care providers in Illinois. J Am Dent Assoc 2007;138(4):519–24.
[29] Glotzer DL, More FG, Phelan J, et al. Introducing a senior course on catastrophic preparedness into the dental school curriculum. J Dent Educ 2006;70(3):225–30.

ELSEVIER
SAUNDERS

Dent Clin N Am 51 (2007) 837–856

THE DENTAL CLINICS OF NORTH AMERICA

The Role of the Dentist at Crime Scenes

Melissa Naiman, MS, EMT-B[a,*],
A. Karl Larsen, Jr, PhD[a,b],
Peter R. Valentin, MSFS[a,c]

[a] *Disaster Emergency Medicine Readiness Training Center, College of Dentistry, University of Illinois at Chicago, 801 S. Paulina Street #569D, M/C 838, Chicago, IL 60622, USA*
[b] *Illinois State Police, Forensic Sciences Command, Forensic Science Center at Chicago, Chicago, IL, USA*
[c] *Connecticut State Police, Major Crime Squad, Litchfield, CT, USA*

The medical response to a mass casualty incident will always be complicated. Providing quality care while understaffed, undersupplied, and possibly operating in an unfamiliar or inhospitable environment is not an easy task. The situation is further complicated when the mass casualty incident is the result of a terrorist act, which forces medical response to occur in conjunction with a federal criminal investigation [1]. Although medical professionals and students commonly receive training on the recognition of terrorist events and appropriate interventions, legal aspects and evidence collection are rarely addressed in depth.

The purpose of the first portion of this article is to provide an overview of legal precedents and forensic techniques that could be applied to a terrorist investigation, with a discussion of specific current and emerging technologies that could be used in the investigation of a chemical, biologic, nuclear/radiologic, or explosive event. The authors hope that this information will assist medical responders to recognize potential physical evidence and persons of interest to become confident that intervention does not necessarily conflict with an investigation [2]. The second portion of this article describes forensic techniques and advances that apply to investigations of the deceased to provide a contrast in the goals and responsibilities of a dental emergency responder and a forensic odontologist, summarized in Tables 1 and 2.

* Corresponding author.
E-mail address: mnaima1@uic.edu (M. Naiman).

doi:10.1016/j.cden.2007.06.004 *dental.theclinics.com*

Table 1
Some goals of dental emergency responders and forensic odontologists

Goals	Dental emergency responder	Forensic odontologist
Personal safety	×	×
Recognize possible evidence in a CBRNE event	×	×
Establish victim identity through personal belongings	×	×
Document chain of custody for all potential evidence	×	×
Provide total body care to victims	×	
Ensure patient well-being above all other priorities	×	
Establish identity through maxillofacial structures		×
Ensure long term evidence fidelity		×

Abbreviation: CBRNE, chemical, biologic, nuclear/radiologic, and explosive.

Dental emergency responder

In light of a nation-wide discussion regarding the role of the oral health community in disaster response [3–10], modifications to the Dental Practice Act were proposed, ratified, and took effect January 1, 2006 [11]. This amendment defined the dental emergency responder as a position within the scope of practice of dentistry in Illinois. Although debate on the specific roles and recommended training continues, in the framework of Illinois, the dental emergency responder is most commonly used to provide total body patient care in one of four roles: (1) care for the worried well (those who are not part of an event but are seeking advice from a medical professional to ensure

Table 2
Possible observations likely to be made by dental emergency responders or forensic odontologists

Observations of interest	Dental emergency responder	Forensic odontologist
Suspected dispersion device on patient body	×	
Blue prints or architectural drawings on patient	×	
Potential explosive device on body of patient	×	
Stage of illness relative to population	×	
Emotional state of patient	×	
Medical records		×
Labeled dentures/tagged molars		×
Database		×
Pathologies		×

the safety of themselves and their family); (2) care for the walking wounded (those in need of minimal medical intervention after an event); (3) triage care (after receiving additional training as part of formalized response team membership); and (4) participants in mass dispensation and mass inoculation response [12]. None of these roles are exclusively filled by dental emergency responders; instead, the dental emergency responder becomes part of a multidisciplinary team dedicated to ensuring the well-being of the community during a terrorist event or public health emergency. Although the examples provided herein are offered with the dental emergency responder (or an equivalent role in another state) in mind, the scenarios could also apply to any medical responder fulfilling the roles defined above.

Pertinent precedents

In any investigation, the bulk of physical evidence is collected by law enforcement professionals or specially trained military units (eg, a National Guard Civilian Support Team). Detailed analysis is performed in a laboratory setting that is determined by the nature of the incident. Nevertheless, there is a chance that medical responders may discover evidence that will be pertinent to an investigation. Specific items that may be of interest to investigators are covered in detail under each scenario. This section provides an overview of case law in Illinois directly related to the act of search and seizure.

Private seizures

The standard for law enforcement officers to perform a search is probable cause; officers receive training specifically related to proper search and seizure protocols and are aware that illegally seized evidence will be excluded from the prosecutor's case in chief [13,14]. This standard does not apply to medical professionals as private citizens. It is common practice to perform a search of a patient's personal belongings if he or she is unconscious or exhibiting an altered mental status to establish identity, medication usage, or the presence of allergies. Should a search of this nature yield evidence, the items may be turned over to law enforcement officials and used by the state for its case in chief, despite the lack of probable cause [15].

Status as a private citizen and medical professional does not allow an individual to perform a search of a patient at the behest of a law enforcement officer if this search would not have been performed otherwise [16]. For example, medical personnel providing care to "worried well" victims that have not been exposed to an agent and are not exhibiting signs of critical injury that would warrant removal of clothing or a search of personal possessions cannot perform a search of a patient at the request of the police. Any evidence obtained through such a scenario in which a law officer encourages a private citizen to perform a search when probable cause is not present will likely be disallowed at trial.

Chain of custody

Once an item of evidence has been seized or is located on a patient, care must be taken to record the whereabouts and access to the item in writing; the more susceptible the item is to contamination or tampering, the more closely it should be monitored [17–19]. For example, an article of clothing with a distinctive logo would be more readily recognizable than a small piece of shrapnel removed from a wound. Medical records can serve as a chain of custody between providers throughout care to establish the time, location, and status for objects of interest that are not removed from the patient on scene but hours or days later [20]. Items that are discovered and collected in the field should be labeled (name of patient, name of practitioner, date, time) and preferably stored in an area with limited public access until they are collected and signed for by a law enforcement officer; inconsistencies in delivery and receipt conditions could lead to the suppression of evidence [21].

Health Information Protection and Accountability Act

The Health Information Protection and Accountability Act (HIPAA) was enacted originally in 1996 [22], with modifications in 2000 and 2002 to ensure the confidentiality of patient information among covered entities, such as health care providers, insurance companies, and health care clearinghouses [23]. During a disaster, the standards of HIPAA still apply; providers should continue to be mindful of protected health information, especially in light of the limited privacy inherent in field response and possible media presence. All medical responders would be considered covered entities, including volunteers, but there are several notable exceptions to accountability and disclosure pertinent to a terrorist attack. Disclosures to law enforcement officials involved in the investigation, to public health authorities involved in surveillance or efforts to avert a serious threat to health and safety, or to protect national security do not require written authorization from an individual patient [24].

Evidence collection and preservation

Overall, medical professionals should attempt to the best of their ability to store evidence in a manner that will facilitate future analysis. First, one should avoid cutting through holes in patient clothing that were created before their arrival for care. Maintaining holes intact will help forensic specialists recreate the scene, corroborate the size and force of an object that penetrated the victim, and give guidance for tests to determine the presence or absence of trace evidence. Cutting through the hole causes permanent distortion to the fabric (especially in the case of knitted fabrics) and can contaminate the surface of the fabric with metal or other debris from the scissors that might not be distinguishable from pertinent evidence. Second, one should avoid sealing items while they are still damp. Wet items may grow mold or mildew that will contaminate the evidence and make further analysis more difficult. If the possibility exists, the item should be allowed to dry before sealing the container. Third, one should avoid the use of plastic bags when possible. Plastic can cause the degradation of biologic and chemical evidence and can lead to a moist environment inside the bag [25]. All evidence, regardless of nature or origin, should be handled with gloved hands to protect it from trace damage (such as fingerprints) and to protect medical professionals from exposure to toxic chemicals or other agents [26]. Although these measures may sound tedious, they have been practiced by sexual assault nurse examiners in hospital settings for over 20 years [27].

Evidence collection summary

Evidence collection does not supersede the responsibility of a medical responder to provide medical care. A medical responder should never hold evidence collection over preservation of life and limb; however, proper collection and storage of evidence discovered on the scene of a mass casualty incident will assist police operations in terms of the viability of detailed analysis and admissibility. By maintaining records of possible evidence, storing evidence in a manner least likely to result in contamination, and submitting evidence to law enforcement officers as expeditiously as possible, medical professionals can do a great service to the investigation of and the victims of a terrorist event.

Forensic techniques and evidence sources in specific scenarios

Intentional man-made events are generally broken down into five major categories: chemical, biologic, nuclear/radiologic, and explosive (CBRNE). Each of these categories can be divided further into specific agents or patient characteristics. To best serve medical responders, for each major category the authors provide a description of standard analysis, an overview of emerging detection and forensic techniques, possible scenarios in which medical professionals may discover evidence, and measures to protect the integrity of the evidence while ensuring personal safety.

Chemical scenario

The specific forensic techniques use in the investigation of a chemical event will vary based on the nature of the agent; however, certain facts will require resolution for the state to build a sufficient case for the prosecution of suspects. The verified agent identity, proof of victim exposure to agents, and the ability of suspects to synthesize and disseminate the agent will be of particular interest to those involved in prosecution.

Preliminary agent identification will likely come as victims present with symptoms associated with toxic exposure (eg, dyspnea, rhinorhea, ocular pain, dizziness, vomiting) [28]. Intelligence related to possible terrorist threats in the area might also support the preliminary agent identification. The support of hazardous material (HAZMAT) teams will provide more information; handheld detectors [29] and manual testing will confirm the presence of an agent class (eg, nerve agent versus sulfur mustard). Improvements in the reliability and range of detectable agents are being explored with the use of different forms of spectrometry (such as Fourier transform infrared spectroscopy), photometry, and chip-based sensors based on carbon nanotubes [30–32].

As part of the detailed analysis, scientists will also note the impurities and precursors found in the sample. Few chemical reactions provide 100% yield in every step; in the Tokyo subway attack, the liquid sampled on the train was only 30% sarin. The other 70% of the substance provided clues as to the synthetic protocol used, allowing law enforcement officials to narrow the search to facilities/business entities that had purchased these chemicals recently [33]. The sophistication of the synthetic model and the purity of the product will also indicate the type of facility and personnel that would likely be associated with the agent production. Examinations of organic and aqueous extractions of samples using instrumentation routinely used in forensic investigations, such as gas chromatography/mass spectrometry and liquid chromatography/mass spectrometry, have proven sufficient to identify most agents, especially when coupled with pre-concentration techniques and tandem mass spectrometry [34,35].

Depending on the agent, identification may be enough to support charges for violating the chemical warfare ban but will not be sufficient to support homicide and battery charges. Most chemical agents are either nonpersistent (vapor) or require wet decontamination. Because life and limb supersede a forensic investigation, samples will not be taken before decontamination or medical intervention, even if personnel were able to take samples on scene. As an alternative to immediate or superficial collection, biophysical changes specific to agent exposure can be determined through blood analysis [36–38]. Raman spectroscopy also shows promise as a noninvasive means to determine exposure to chemical and biologic agents [39].

At the time of an attack, it is highly likely that intelligence gathering will have narrowed the field of suspects. Through interrogation and investigative work, it is also possible that a facility or dissemination device will be located. The analytical techniques and instrumentation discussed previously can be applied to confirm the presence of chemical agents on equipment. Precursors, solvents, and equipment consistent with the suspected synthetic model will likely be present in the facility where the agent was manufactured [33].

Chemical events are particularly dangerous to medical responders, especially for those operating in the "cold zone." Many chemical agents can be absorbed through the skin (or latex gloves), leaving responders vulnerable to secondary contamination. By the time a dental responder is on scene, the nature of the agent will be at least preliminarily confirmed, and the manner of decontamination will have been decided. With this in mind, observing a patient's attempt to avoid decontamination (which will require removal of clothing) should be considered highly suspicious, and law enforcement officials should be notified of this behavior. If when monitoring patients triaged as minimally injured, several patients exhibit a sudden onset of more severe symptoms simultaneously, the medical responder should notify medical team leaders and law enforcement. The sudden onset may be caused by a secondary device or by proximity to the dissemination device. In both instances, the authorities should be notified, and all personnel should prepare to undergo decontamination measures. If the agent is persistent, the medical responder should report any objects found in the patient's possession or in the treatment area that appear oily or greasy but should not attempt to handle the item, even with gloved hands.

Biologic agents

The investigation of a biologic agent is the most challenging CBRNE event. Although an outbreak of an unusual nature (such as smallpox) would trigger an immediate response and investigation, most biologic agents act slowly within a population, and patients present with nondescript ailments in many locations over an extended period of time (days or weeks as opposed to minutes or hours in a chemical attack). The core questions of agent identity, patient exposure, and agent production require investigation.

In the best case scenario, agents will be detected before an infection occurs. The persistence of biologic agents and the necessity of relatively high concentrations of biologic agents for infection to occur are used to the advantage of law enforcement and public health officials. Various federal efforts to create sentinel detectors, such as the Biological Aerosol Sentry and Information System (BASIS), BioWatch, and Automated Biological Agent Testing System (ABATS) [29] aim to provide identification of agents as they are released into the environment through continuous sampling at a static location; however, these technologies rely on the airborne presence of the agent, which may not occur in cases of food-borne dissemination [40].

Currently, sentinels are not ubiquitous; therefore, a real possibility remains that the first warning of an attack will occur when citizens become infected. Agent identity will initially be established through common histologic procedures performed at hospitals, public health laboratories, or specialized facilities [41,42]. Analytical techniques are being refined to offer faster and more accurate agent characterization that can be used for any type of agent and to more readily recognize hoaxes [43–45]. Microchip-based technologies allow for simultaneous detection of multiple agents in the field and clinical settings [46,47].

The prevalence of genetic engineering may also contribute to a delayed recognition of a biologic attack [48]. Techniques widely used in academic and commercial settings allow scientists to control the genetic properties and abilities of bacterial and viral agents, meaning that an agent could "look" like salmonella during screening but actually contain the genetic ability to produce a more virulent toxin. Projects to map bacterial and viral genomes are underway to provide baseline information about genetic differences between and among strains that are currently found in the environment so that the future release of a laboratory cultured agent will be more readily apparent [40,49,50].

Unlike chemical agents, the production of biologic agents does not require regulated chemical precursors. The equipment and chemicals necessary to replicate or modify a bacteria or virus have many benign uses and are ubiquitous in biologic and genetic laboratories, enhancing the possibility of "dual use" facilities [51]. Several businesses are devoted solely to the creation of DNA sequences to order and do not always screen these sequences against the DNA sequences of known biologic agents; therefore, the possibility exists that a major part of production did not even occur within a facility [52]. Nevertheless, intelligence suggesting that this method was used to orchestrate a biologic attack would allow law enforcement to trace involved parties through billing records of a sequencing company. Rather than focusing on the specific location or ability to produce the parent agent, a link to the equipment used in the replication of the agent might be established. DNA analysis of samples found in a suspected facility could be compared with the DNA analysis of samples taken from the scene and from victims, and statistical models derived from genome mapping projects could allow probabilities of association to be extrapolated, much in the same manner that DNA analysis of bodily fluids can yield a probability of association with an individual [50].

A medical provider may contribute to an investigation in two likely ways: (1) by recognizing and reporting a person of interest or (2) by recognizing a device that was part of the dissemination of the agent. During any sort of epidemic (natural or intentional), populations are affected at different times and at different rates; a patient presenting with a more developed infection than anyone else in the area is a person of interest. This individual may have come into contact with the agent before anyone else in the community (perhaps as a result of travel) or may have had involvement in the synthesis or dissemination of the agent. In both cases, this person will assist public health and law enforcement authorities in pinpointing the origins of the outbreak and will provide useful information in the case of an outbreak. The second possibility is the discovery of a dissemination device in the possession of a patient. Items such as vials, medicine droppers, test tubes, and other containers would be of interest to law enforcement officials, particularly if these containers were concealed but provided easy access, such as being taped to the wrist. Another item of interest would be architectural plans, especially if they include details of a heating, ventilating, and air conditioning system [53]. Handling items potentially contaminated with biologic agents should be performed while using the recommended personal protective equipment associated with the particular agent.

Nuclear/radiologic event

A radiologic event will require immediate evacuation (much like a chemical event) and the intervention of specially trained teams, such as the National Guard Weapons of Mass Destruction Civilian Support Team, the Department of Energy Nuclear Emergency Support Teams, and the Environmental Protection Agency [54], in detection, characterization, and recovery efforts. If recently suggested guidelines are adopted, an area of 500 m (approximately 0.31 miles) will be evacuated and considered the "hot" zone where radiation levels are considered too high to operate without appropriate protection and medical oversight [55]. Information discovered by these teams could be used at the launch of a police investigation. For example, the specific isotope discovered on scene will indicate whether the material was likely to have been derived from industrial or medical instrumentation and will lead to the cross-check of those facilities for reports of stolen or damaged equipment [55]. Detector technology based on neutron generation and gamma ray spectra interpretation offers the ability to characterize unexploded ordnance [56].

As the threat of radiologic exposure diminishes, information about the device can be sought similar to the investigation of an explosion, especially in the case of a radiologic dispersion device or "dirty bomb." Emerging technologies are capable of detecting and classifying explosives from a distance, making it possible for information to be gathered while minimizing the chance of injury. Again, forensic scientists will focus on the explosives and the contaminants to link the device with a facility and a perpetrator.

The most probable circumstance for medical volunteer involvement would be in response to a radiologic dispersion device. If a patient presents with symptoms associated with high levels of radiation exposure but shows no sign of trauma or gross external contamination or if he or she presents with only burns to the hands or forearms, the patient would be a person of interest to law enforcement because they may have been involved in the preparation or transport of the device. Patients close to the explosion site may receive penetrating injuries from shrapnel. Facilities on scene and operating procedures may not allow for the removal of the foreign body, but a note on the nature of the shrapnel, patient information, and destination hospital (if known) would be useful to the investigation. If the foreign body is removed (if it is blocking the airway), provider information, the time, date, and patient information should be noted on the bag and the item placed away from traffic flow until law enforcement officials are able to retrieve it. In the radiologic dispersion device scenario, the amount of particulate matter on a single piece of shrapnel is not likely to cause a health risk.

Explosive events

Bombings are the most common form of terrorist action to date. Hundreds of events have occurred internationally causing countless fatalities and casualties [57]. As a result, law enforcement agencies are relatively prepared for the necessary analyses following an explosive event; most forensic laboratories have sections devoted to arson and explosive investigations [58,59]. Some police forces cross-train officers in urban search and rescue to allow forensic investigators early access to the crime scene in the safest manner possible. As is true in the other scenarios, the goal of the forensic investigation is to characterize the agent (through recreation of the device and the chemical composition of the explosives), link the agent to an individual or group, and prove that an individual or group planted the device in a specific location.

To prove the existence of an explosive device (as opposed to an accidental explosion), investigators seek evidence of the four required components of an improvised explosive device: a power source, initiators, explosives, and switches. A fifth component, which is not necessary but can provide useful information, is fragmentation and shrapnel such as ball bearings, nuts, and screws included as part of the device to inflict greater damage and increase the likelihood of secondary blast injuries. Bringing these components together can give officers an idea of the level of sophistication of the device and the level of training of the offenders and can provide a possible connection between crimes. For example, the use of home-manufactured rather than commercially machined screws was a trademark of explosives in the Unabomber cases, and the use of a Big Ben alarm clock was consistent among all of the devices planted by Eric Rudolph (the Olympic Park bomber). Also, if several devices were used in the same attack, evidence of these necessary components would confirm the number of devices used and whether specific design characteristics were shared among the devices.

Characterization of the actual explosive will begin with an examination of the physical characteristics of the device fragments. Low explosives deflagrate, that is, they propagate energy through thermal conductivity; therefore, the discovery of fragments that are warped or charred would be indicative of a low explosive. High explosives detonate, which is the propagation of energy through a pressure wave at supersonic speeds; fragments that have sharp edges and limited signs of heat exposure would indicate the possible use of a high explosive [60,61]. If physical components are not immediately recovered, surrounding structures and damaged objects can be swabbed and tested for the presence of explosive residue. Currently, colormetric tests are employed to determine whether to sample an area or object for more specific analysis. Such tests rely on a chemical reaction between the explosive and an introduced agent that results in a color change [61]. Studies of the use of photoluminscent techniques that use laser excitation to improve visualization in the field have been developed and are undergoing validation and testing [62]. In specialized laboratory settings, explosive identification may also be achieved through re-crystallization and observation under polarized light [63].

Some of the handheld monitors used for chemical detection can also detect the presence of explosives [30]; however, more sensitive and accurate instrumentation based on Raman spectrometry is emerging that is capable of detecting explosive mixtures at a distance [64]. Neutron interrogation devices have demonstrated the ability to characterize explosives (and other substances) by reading the gamma ray signatures released by an object following excitation by neutrons released by the detector [56]. This testing is especially useful in the determination of the fill of unexploded or buried devices [65].

Further confirmation can be achieved with laboratory-based analysis, which is made necessary by the fact that most improvised explosives are derived from commonly used, commercially available products with benign uses. For example, a nitrate-based fertilizer mixed with diesel fuel creates an explosive material (ammonium nitrate fuel oil). The presence of nitrates or the presence of diesel fuel is insufficient to definitively characterize the nature of the explosive; both substances could be detected by chance in a given area. Analytical techniques that reveal more information about the specific structure or molecule complex are more useful in characterizing explosives [66]. Sensitivity is further improved with concentration techniques such a solid phase extraction [67] before analysis, as well as the use of artificial neuronal networks, a form of enhanced software to modulate the separation conditions according to the specific needs of the sample [68]. Recently, success has been reported in extracting DNA from skin cells left on the surface of exploded pipe bombs; therefore, genetic analysis could also prove that an individual handled a specific device [69].

The aim of the primary investigation of a suspect is to connect the individual or a group with the explosives used in an event. Police officers will likely use preliminary techniques on scene, such as colormetric tests, to determine the presence of explosives and will use the results as probable cause to detain a suspect pending further investigation. Explosive residues are readily collected from nonporous surfaces, skin, and fabric. Studies have shown that hair has the ability to concentrate vapors from some military explosives and that concentrations can be linked to exposure time and still be traced after washing or environmental exposure [70,71]. In the laboratory setting, characteristics of trace elements associated with the explosive, such as sulfur, can be analyzed to associate the explosive material with a suspect or may be found in the suspect's possession (even in trace form) with explosive material recovered from the scene [72].

The nature of an explosive event provides the greatest opportunity for a medical responder to recover evidence or identify persons of interest.

The most dangerous situation would be the discovery of an undetonated device on the body of a patient. This situation might occur in a suicide bombing in which multiple bombers planned to attack a site, one or more perpetrators carried devices that did not detonate, and the suspects sustained injury as a result of the proximate blast, or if the device was intended to detonate upon removal from the patient by medical personnel. In the event of such a discovery, one should notify law enforcement immediately. Do not attempt to remove the device or move the patient any more than absolutely necessary. Evacuate the surrounding area rather than attempting to move the device (or the patient it is attached to). Other persons of interest may be less severely wounded patients who act nervous rather than panicked, particularly if the individual seems focused on police activities. Law enforcement officials may not be readily available for interrogation, but a detailed description of the individual including identifying characteristics and contact information should be provided to investigators, along with any transport information.

Penetrative injuries of varying severity are common in bombings [73]; recorded injuries range from hardware to bone fragments [74] from a suicide bomber. Because fragmentation evidence can be useful in device reconstruction or trace analysis, police knowledge of the removal of such fragments from patients is useful. Fragments associated directly with the device are important; objects that resemble batteries, springs, electronics (eg, wires, transistors, microchips, cellular phone components), or plastic tubing should be noted. If the items are removed in the field, one should package and store shrapnel following the guidelines presented previously, making sure to wear gloves and a mask to prevent DNA contamination. In the more likely circumstance that the patient is transported with the shrapnel still embedded, the medical responder should make note of the patient's name, identifying characteristics, the nature of the shrapnel, and the transport hospital (if known) and should provide this information to law enforcement officials.

In an explosive event that creates extreme structural damage, clothing removed from patients evacuated from the scene could be of use. Evidence collection will always run secondary to engineering concerns such as structure stability. The ability to start the investigation by conducting an initial analysis on articles of clothing will save a great deal of time, because safety concerns may disallow evidence collection from the explosion site for hours or days. One should store items of clothing as described earlier.

Role of dentists in mass disaster forensics

Forensic interest in mass disasters centers on determination of the cause of the disaster and identification of the victims rather than preservation of life and limb. Historically, methods have included simple recognition, use of fingerprints, dental records, and skeletal identification using radiologic or anthropologic means. DNA analysis has become an essential tool in the analysis of samples in cases in which severe fragmentation of victims is involved. These methods in concert have led to the successful identification of thousands of victims of disasters such as earthquakes, floods, tsunami, or terrorist attacks. Each of these methods of identification has strengths and weaknesses that must be taken into account when evidence is collected. Proper preservation and storage of evidence is critical if analysis is to be accomplished in a reliable, efficient manner. Coordination of all analytical teams is also essential to provide a flow of evidence from section to section; all must work in concert to perform a task that can be of monumental proportion.

Evidence protocols

Evidence processing, no matter what the disaster, is crucial to maintaining integrity of the collected evidence so that analytical results will stand up to scrutiny in the courts and provide closure for the families of the victims. This collection begins with recovery of the evidence and processing in the site for analysis; without the time constraints imposed by the responsibility of patient care, evidence documentation is more rigorous. Each item of possible evidentiary value will undergo the following: (1) photography; (2) logging of personal effects, if any; (3) fingerprinting if possible; (4) jaw resection and dental radiology; (5) full body radiology; (6) dental examination and charting; (7) autopsy; (8) embalming; (9) body preparation for shipping; and (10) casketing and shipping [75]. The forensic odontology team will be highly involved in steps 4 to 6; their work will be suspect without proper in-processing and documentation.

Forensic odontology

In many instances, such as when victims are severely burned, traditional forensic techniques do not provide conclusive means of identification. Pathologic conditions noted in dental records, treatments, and prosthetic devices may survive fires when identifying markings and DNA may not. Dental records are among the most readily available ante mortem information that can be accessed by disaster emergency response teams. As such, forensic odontology continues to be a crucial element in nearly all mass disasters whether natural, accidental, or intentional. At the onset of a disaster, various teams of dentists will be established to start collecting ante mortem data based on lists of missing persons, a task that relies heavily on the nature of victims (eg, military versus civilian). Once these records have been compiled, forensic odontologists can begin comparisons between remains and ante mortem records. Traditionally, overlays [76] have been used in many disaster situations, even before the 1980s. These overlay procedures have been simplified with time and still serve local coroner or medical examiner offices that may not have the volume or resources to maintain a database; however, the number of victims in a mass disaster situation makes simple comparison unacceptable. Overlays have given way to computerized matching software

[75,77,78]. Data comparison systems such as computer-assisted postmortem identification (CAPMI) [75], WinID [78], Plass [79], and DAVID [77] software have enabled rapid entry of ante mortem records and post mortem data into a database capable of completing rapid comparison of huge amounts of data. Each program has allowed new levels of detail and greater operator control leading to increased suggested match accuracy; however, all suggested matches are verified by members of the mass disaster team.

Other information beyond the description of dentition can be used in the forensic odontology field, such as labeled dental prostheses. Victims possessing all or most of their dentition have physical characteristics necessary for their identification, whereas those missing all of their teeth lack such information. Identification from prosthetics has been around since the 1800s. Markings on prosthetic devices should be able to establish the identity of the patient or victim, be easily and quickly applied, and be fire resistant or placed in such a manner that they are protected by the tongue. The marking should not interfere with the function of the device and be unobtrusive, and the appearance should be acceptable to the patient [80]. Some of the simplest marking techniques involve surface marks inscribed by scalpels, pencil marks that are covered by dental polymer, and inscribing the cast from which the device was made. More recently, markings have been enclosed in the prosthetic device using polymethyl methacrylate to ensure permanency. Metal identification bands have been enclosed in compartments within the device, which are completely invisible when completed and cosmetically appealing but readily recognizable during radiologic examination. Radiofrequency identification (RFID) tags have been developed that are small enough to be implanted into a prosthesis [80] or a prepared molar [81]. This technology originally served the veterinary field but is easily transferred to human use. Identification would be accomplished through the use of an interrogator that triggers a power surge in the RFID chip which responds by providing information to the reader. This method could, if implemented, ease the work involved in the identification of victims of a mass disaster; however, there will be some time lapse before such devices are frequently seen in the overall population.

Forensic dentistry has provided victim identification in many different scenarios involving many different types and numbers of victims. As the result of a major highway accident in Spain in 1996, 28 victims were processed, and 16 of the victims were identified through dental records. The remaining 12 were not owing to extensive destruction of the dentition by fire or a lack of dental records [82].

In another example, the USS Iowa explosion, 45 of 47 victims were identified through dental comparison either alone or in conjunction with fingerprint matching [83]. Because the victims were active duty military personnel, high quality, up-to-date dental records were easily available, providing optimum circumstances for dental comparisons to be completed. The crash of Arrow Airways Flight 950 near Gander Airport in Newfoundland, Canada, provides a contrast to the ideal operational conditions in the USS Iowa investigation. As in the previous case, forensic odontology contributed to a significant number of the nearly 250 US Army personnel identifications; however, unlike in the USS Iowa explosion, the servicemen were carrying their medical and dental records during the flight. The Armed Forces Institute of Pathology was charged with the identification of the victims. The team consisted of 23 armed forces dental officers and 16 support staff. One subgroup of these personnel, the dental registrar, was charged with the receipt, inventory, and custody of all obtained medical records. Because the primary dental records were mostly fragmented or destroyed in the crash, records were obtained from civilian sources [75]. Privacy considerations slowed the access to medical records of individuals; fortunately, records can be transferred in cases of disaster when the third party is in the medical field and involved in the identification process, an exemption that still holds under current HIPAA regulations.

Two aspects of this case were of importance to the future of forensic identification using dental records. First, protocols now prohibit military personnel from carrying medical records with them during transport. Second, this case was the first to use CAPMI to assist the comparison of dental records [75]. This system was the first to gain popularity and widespread use in forensic identification because it allowed for simultaneous comparisons at multiple sites.

In the Asian tsunami of 2004, dental records contributed to nearly 85% of the identifications [79]. The tsunami provides an example of the problems that can arise in a forensic response to a mass disaster. This case involved over 200,000 dead and injured persons. Nearly 60 nations were represented in the victims, and ten nations were affected by the disaster. Disaster relief came from around the world, and victim identification teams were sent from more than 20 countries, necessitating the adoption of universal protocols before evidence collection and analysis. The standard operating procedures for all steps of the identification process, including ante mortem record requests, fingerprint identification, forensic pathology and odontology, and DNA analysis, had to be agreed upon. Interpol took the lead in trying to coordinate data and institute standard operating procedures for physical evidence, but the legalities involved in obtaining medical records had to be negotiated. Interpol also issued guidelines to help with the ante mortem records collection. The Interpol Victim Identification Guide, section 6.3.2.2, required all nations with possible missing citizens to provide all necessary records in an expedient manner; however, some countries took a conservative approach and gave estimated numbers of missing citizens, whereas others reported the numbers of citizens reported missing and presumed dead. This response inflated the number of records thought to be necessary in the identification process. The Interpol Victim Identification Guide also required original records in section 4.5.2.5; however, worldwide, the records that were sent varied greatly in quality, and many copies were substituted for original records. Even more crucial were the procedures necessary for the collection and preservation of evidence and the maintenance of the chain of custody of the evidence which would be used in the identification; speed was necessary due to the climate and the rapid decomposition of the bodies [79].

As is true for a medical response, forensic odontology and mass disasters involve the use of personnel other than dentists. Support personnel such as dental hygienists have been trained to participate in the identification process. They have assumed roles in the ante mortem processing team, the radiologic processing team, and the post mortem team. These tasks require training in chain of custody techniques, in record keeping for forensic documentation, and in quality management guidelines [84]. More personnel involved in the process can spread the work and relieve stress. The observed effects on health care professionals participating in mass disaster work have been documented to include distress while participating but also relief and satisfaction by making a positive impact in a disaster situation. Support gained through the other professionals in the work group adds to the positive feelings that can be derived through successful work in a mass disaster [85]. Further documentation indicates that persons who participate in mock disaster drills feel they are better prepared to participate in authentic events [86]. Additional personnel in conjunction with increased training opportunities should help reduce the stress on involved personnel and aid in faster analysis times.

Summary

As the role of the oral health professional as a medical responder becomes more widely accepted throughout the country, the probability of a dental emergency responder responding to a terrorist event (a de facto crime scene) will increase. As part of continuing education, oral health professionals interested in pursuing a role in disaster response should seek out opportunities to enhance their knowledge of rules of evidence in the states in which they practice and obtain knowledge of operating procedures and technical capacities specific to their city, county, and state. This knowledge will help the dental emergency responder distinguish physical evidence that is most likely to be of analytical value.

The first priority of the medical responder is to provide quality care to the victims of a mass casualty incident; no piece of evidence is more valuable than life and limb. Nevertheless, there are many scenarios in which evidence collection does not conflict with patient care. Responders are not responsible for the interrogation or detention of anyone and should not attempt either action, but recording as much information as possible about suspicious individuals or patients who may be in possession of physical evidence (even if it is embedded in the patient's body) will greatly assist the investigation. Medical personnel should remember that patient information provided to law enforcement officials during the course of an investigation is exempt from HIPAA oversights and does not require written authorization.

Investigators rely on the cooperation of many community members throughout an investigation; in a mass casualty incident, cooperation with the medical community is invaluable.

In providing information on investigative techniques, the authors hope to simplify the process of recognizing, collecting, and storing evidence during a mass casualty incident. Prosecution following a terrorist event is a meaningful part of the recovery phase, and forensic evidence will likely have a strong role in any legal action. By following the guidelines presented herein, medical responders will be able to minimize the risk of contamination and of evidence suppression due to a flawed chain of command.

Law enforcement and medical response provide two vital functions during a mass casualty incident. Both professions should continue to remain aware of standards and guidelines that affect practice to remain sensitive to the needs surrounding a given function. This awareness will enhance mutual respect and cooperation, which will, in turn, positively impact the overall response and recovery in the event of a terrorist attack.

References

[1] Representatives UHo. 18 USC § 2331.

[2] Du J, Mont DP. The doctor's dilemma: caregiving and medicolegal evidence collection. Med Law 2004;23(3):515–29.

[3] Alfano MC. Bioterrorism response. J Am Dent Assoc 2003;134(3):278–80.

[4] Assael LA. Readiness and response: the oral and maxillofacial surgeon's role in disaster. J Oral Maxillofac Surg 2005;63(11):1565–6.

[5] Chmar JE, Ranney RR, Guay AH, et al. Incorporating bioterrorism training into dental education: report of ADA-ADEA terrorism and mass casualty curriculum development workshop. J Dent Educ 2004;68(11):1196–9.

[6] Downes EJ. We've got the skills. Let's use them. N Y State Dent J 2003;69(5):24.

[7] Morlang WM. Dentistry's vital role in disaster preparedness. J Calif Dent Assoc 1996;24(5): 63–6.

[8] Weber CR. Dentistry's role in biodefense. PA Dent J (Harrisb) 2003;70(5):32–4.

[9] Guay AH. Dentistry's response to bioterrorism: a report of a consensus workshop. J Am Dent Assoc 2002;133(9):1181–7.

[10] Research NIoDaC. Dentistry's role in responding to bioterrorism and other catastrophic events. Available at: http://www.nidcr.nih.gov/NewsAndReports/ReportsPresentation/DentistrysRoleInRespondingToBioterrorismAndOtherCatastrophicEvents.htm. Accessed August 21, 2006.

[11] Illinois general assembly. Public Act 094-0409. Available at: http://www.ilga.gov/legislation/publicacts/fulltext.asp?name = 094-0409&GA = 094. Accessed March 11, 2007.

[12] Colvard MD, Lampiris LN, Cordell GA, et al. The dental emergency responder: expanding the scope of dental practice. J Am Dent Assoc 2006;137(4):468–73.

[13] Patrick H. O'Donnell TDN, Oscar E. Carlstrom. People v. Scalisi, 324 Ill. 131, 154 N.E. 715. Vol No. 17745; 1926.

[14] Thomas J. McCormick JEC. People v. Dalpe, 371 Ill. 607; 21 N.E.2d 756. Vol No. 25098; 1939.

[15] People v. Radcliff. 305 Ill. App. 3d 493; 712 N.E.2d 424; 1999.

[16] People v. Flagg. Vol. 217 Ill. App. 3d 655, 577 N.E. 2d 815, 160 Ill. Dec. 490: Illinois 5th District; 1991.

[17] McCormick CT. McCormick's handbook of the law of evidence (Hornbook series). 2nd edition. St. Paul (MN):West Pub Co; 1972.

[18] Ralph Ruebner DM, Bernard Carey. People v. Valentin. 66 Ill. App. 3d 488; 384 N.E.2d 67; 1978 Ill. App. Vol No. 77-1648: First District, First Division; 1978.
[19] Robert Weiner TLF, C. Joseph Cavanagh. People v. Rhoades. 74 Ill. App. 3d 247; 392 N.E.2d 923. Vol No. 15326; 1979.
[20] Robert Agostinelli MR, David DeDoncker. People v. Rogers. 42 Ill. App. 3d 499; 356 N.E.2d 413. Vol No. 75-55: Appellate Court of Illinois, Third District; 1976.
[21] Allan Ackerman FFC, Albert Kennedy. People v. Woessner. 132 Ill. App. 2d 58; 268 N.E.2d 508. Vol No. 70-81; 1971.
[22] Health Insurance Portability and Accountability Act of 1996. Public Law 104-191. Available at: http://www.cms.hhs.gov/HIPAAGenInfo/Downloads/HIPAALaw.pdf. Accessed March 13, 2007.
[23] 45 C.F.R. § 164.512. HIPAA Act for disclosures; 2000.
[24] Cole LJ, Fleisher LD. Update on HIPAA privacy: are you ready? Genet Med 2003;5(3): 183–6.
[25] Nayduch D. Trauma wound management. Wound Care Management 1999;34(4):895–906.
[26] McGillivray B. The role of Victorian emergency nurses in the collection and preservation of forensic evidence: a review of the literature. Accid Emerg Nurs 2005;13(2):95–100.
[27] Evans MMRN, Stagner PARN. Maintaining the chain of custody: evidence handling in forensic cases. AORN J 2003;78(4):563–4, 566–567, 569.
[28] Kenar L, Karayilanoglu T, Eryilmaz M, et al. Chemical release at the airport and lessons learned from the medical perspective. J Hazard Mater 2007;144(1–2):396–9.
[29] Fitch JP, Raber E, Imbro DR. Technology challenges in responding to biological or chemical attacks in the civilian sector. 10.1126/science.1085922. Science 2003;302(5649):1350–4.
[30] Davis G. CBRNE-chemical detection equipment. 2006. Available at: http://www.emedicine.com/emerg/topic924.htm. Accessed January 22, 2007.
[31] Robinson JA, Snow ES, Badescu SC, et al. Role of defects in single-walled carbon nanotube chemical sensors. Nano Lett 2006;6(8):1747–51.
[32] Sadik OA, Wanekaya AK, Andreescu S. Advances in analytical technologies for environmental protection and public safety. J Environ Monit 2004;6(6):513–22.
[33] Seto Y. The sarin gas attack in Japan and the related forensic investigation. Synthesis 2001 Summer. Available at: http://www.opcw.org/synthesis/html/s6/p14prt.html. Accessed March 13, 2007.
[34] D'Agostino PA, Hancock JR, Provost LR. Determination of sarin, soman and their hydrolysis products in soil by packed capillary liquid chromatography-electrospray mass spectrometry. J Chromatogr A 2001;912(2):291–9.
[35] Mei-ling L, Hai-ling X, Da-nian X, et al. Identification of certain chemical agents in complex organic solutions by gas chromatography/tandem mass spectrometry. J Mass Spectrom 2006;41(11):1453–8.
[36] Tsuge K, Seto Y. Analysis of organophosphorus compound adducts of serine proteases by liquid chromatography-tandem mass spectrometry. J Chromatogr B Analyt Technol Biomed Life Sci 2002;776(1):79–88.
[37] Tsuge K, Seto Y. Detection of human butyrylcholinesterase-nerve gas adducts by liquid chromatography-mass spectrometric analysis after in gel chymotryptic digestion. J Chromatogr B Analyt Technol Biomed Life Sci 2006;838(1):21–30.
[38] Noort D, Hulst AG, de Jong LP, et al. Alkylation of human serum albumin by sulfur mustard in vitro and in vivo: mass spectrometric analysis of a cysteine adduct as a sensitive biomarker of exposure. Chem Res Toxicol 1999;12(8):715–21.
[39] Notingher I, Green C, Dyer C, et al. Discrimination between ricin and sulphur mustard toxicity in vitro using Raman spectroscopy. J R Soc Interface 2004;1(1):79–90.
[40] Cebula TA, Jackson SA, Brown EW, et al. Chips and SNPs, bugs and thugs: a molecular sleuthing perspective. J Food Prot 2005;68(6):1271–84.
[41] Control CfD. Laboratory network for biological terrorism. 2006. Available at: http://www.bt.cdc.gov/lrn/biological.asp. Accessed January 22, 2007.

[42] Control CfD. Spot tests of selected organisms. Available at: http://www.bt.cdc.gov/documents/PPTResponse/table4spottests.pdf. Accessed January 22, 2007.
[43] Hybl JD, Tysk SM, Berry SR, et al. Laser-induced fluorescence-cued, laser-induced breakdown spectroscopy biological-agent detection. Appl Opt 2006;45:8806–14.
[44] Wilkes JG, Raffi F, Sutherland JB, et al. Pyrolysis mass spectrometry for distinguishing potential hoax materials from bioterror agents. Rapid Commun Mass Spectrom 2006; 20(16):2383–6.
[45] Tomaso H, Scholz HC, Neubauer H, et al. Real-time PCR using hybridization probes for the rapid and specific identification of *Francisella tularensis* subspecies *tularensis*. Mol Cell Probes 2007;21(1):12–6.
[46] Chinowsky TM, Soelberg SD, Baker P, et al. Portable 24-analyte surface plasmon resonance instruments for rapid, versatile biodetection. Biosensors and Bioelectronics 2007;22(9–10): 2268–75.
[47] Koch S, Wolf H, Danapel C, et al. Optical flow-cell multichannel immunosensor for the detection of biological warfare agents. Biosens Bioelectron 2000;14(10–11): 779–84.
[48] Rappert B. Biological weapons, genetics and social analysis: emerging responses, emerging issues. I. New Genet Soc 2003;22(2):169–81.
[49] Budowle B, Schutzer SE, Einseln A, et al. Building microbial forensics as a response to bioterrorism. Science 2003;301(5641):1852–3.
[50] Budowle B, Johnson M, Fraser C, et al. Genetic analysis and attribution of microbial forensics evidence. Crit Rev Microbiol 2005;31(4):233–54.
[51] Franz DR, Zaitchuk R. Biological terrorism: understanding the threat, preparation, and medical response. Dis Mon 2002;48(8):493–564.
[52] Boutin P. Biowar for dummies. 2006 Available at: http://paulboutin.weblogger.com/stories/storyReader$1439. Accessed January 22, 2007.
[53] CIDRAP. History, likely agents, perpetrators, and dissemination. 2002. Available at: http://www.cidrap.umn.edu/cidrap/content/bt/bioprep/biofacts/bioterr-overview.html. Accessed January 22, 2007.
[54] Remick AL, Crapo JL, Woodruff CR. US national response assets for radiological incidents [article]. Health Phys 2005;89(5):471–84.
[55] Musolino SV, Harper FT. Emergency response guidance for the first 48 hours after the outdoor detonation of an explosive radiological dispersal device [article]. Health Phys 2006; 90(4):377–85.
[56] Strellis D, Gozani T. Classifying threats with a 14-MeV neutron interrogation system. Appl Radiat Isot 2005;63(5–6):799–803.
[57] Crabtree J. Terrorist homicide bombings: a primer for preparation. J Burn Care Res 2006; 27(5):576–88.
[58] Yallop HJ. Breaking offences with explosives–the techniques of the criminal and the scientist. J Forensic Sci Soc 1974;14(2):99–102.
[59] Beveridge AD, Payton SF, Audette RJ, et al. Systematic analysis of explosive residues. J Forensic Sci 1975;20(3):431–54.
[60] Saferstein R. Forensic science handbook, Vol. I. 2nd edition. Englewood Cliffs (NJ):Prentice Hall; 2002.
[61] Saferstein R. Criminalistics: an introduction to forensic science. 8th edition. Englewood Cliffs (NJ):Prentice Hall; 2004.
[62] Menzel ER, Bouldin KK, Murdock RH. Trace explosives detection by photoluminescence. Scientific World Journal 2004;4:55–66.
[63] McCrone WC, McCrone LB, Delly JG. Polarized light microscopy. 16th edition. Chicago (IL) :Microscope Publications Ltd; 2005.
[64] Carter JC, Angel SM, Lawrence-Snyder M, et al. Standoff detection of high explosive materials at 50 meters in ambient light conditions using a small Raman instrument. Appl Spectrosc 2005;59:769–75.

[65] Steward S, Forsht D. Use of nuclear techniques to determine the fill of found unexploded ordnance. Appl Radiat Isot 2005;63(5–6):795–7.

[66] De Tata D, Collins P, Campbell N. The identification of the emulsifier component of emulsion explosives by liquid chromatography-mass spectrometry. J Forensic Sci 2006;51(2): 303–7.

[67] Perr JM, Furton KG, Almirall JR. Solid phase microextraction ion mobility spectrometer interface for explosive and taggant detection. J Sep Sci 2005;28(2):177–83.

[68] Casamento S, Kwok B, Roux C, et al. Optimization of the separation of organic explosives by capillary electrophoresis with artificial neural networks. J Forensic Sci 2003;48(5): 1075–83.

[69] Esslinger KJ, Siegel JA, Spillane H, et al. Using STR analysis to detect human DNA from exploded pipe bomb devices. J Forensic Sci 2004;49(3):481–4.

[70] Oxley JC, Smith JL, Kirschenbaum LJ, et al. Accumulation of explosives in hair. J Forensic Sci 2005;50(4):826–31.

[71] Sanders KP, Marshall M, Oxley JC, et al. Preliminary investigation into the recovery of explosives from hair. Sci Justice 2002;42(3):137–42.

[72] Bradley KS. Determination of elemental sulfur in explosives and explosive residues by gas chromatography-mass spectrometry. J Forensic Sci 2005;50(1):96–103.

[73] Arnold JL, Halpern P, Tsai M-C, et al. Mass casualty terrorist bombings: a comparison of outcomes by bombing type. Ann Emerg Med 2004;43(2):263–73.

[74] Hiss J, Freund M, Motro U, et al. The medico-legal investigation of the El Aqsah Intifada. Isr Med Assoc J 2002;4(7):549–53.

[75] Brannon RB, Morlang WM, Smith BC. The Gander disaster: dental identification in a mass tragedy. Journal of Forensic Sciences 2003;48(6):1331–5.

[76] Jones GF. A simple overlay system for data comparison in dental examination. Journal of Forensic Sciences 1998;33(1):254–9.

[77] Clement JG, Winship V, Ceddia J, et al. New software for computer-assisted dental data matching in disaster victim identification and long-term missing persons investigations: DAVID Web. Forensic Science International 2006;159(1 Supp):S24–9.

[78] Lewis C. WinID2 versus CAPMI4: two computer-assisted dental identification systems. J Forensic Sci 2002;47(3):536–8.

[79] DeValck E. Major incident response: collecting ante-mortem data. Forensic Sci Int 2006; 159(Suppl 1):S15–9.

[80] Richmond R, Pretty IA. Contemporary methods of labeling dental prostheses–a review of the literature. J Forensic Sci 2006;51(5):1120–6.

[81] Thevissen PW, Poelman G, DeCooman M, et al. Implantation of an RFID-tag into human molars to reduce hard forensic identification labor. Part I. Working principle. Forensic Sci Int 2006;159(Suppl 1):S33–9.

[82] Valenzuela A, Martin-de las Heras S, Marques T, et al. The application of dental methods of identification to human burn victims in a mass disaster. Int J Legal Med 2000;113:236–9.

[83] Brannon RB, Morlang WM. The USS Iowa disaster: success of the forensic dental team. Journal of Forensic Sciences 2004;49(5):1067–8.

[84] Brannon RB, Connick CM. The role of the dental hygienist in mass disasters. J Forensic Sci 2000;45(2):381–3.

[85] Webb DA, Sweet D, Pretty IA. The emotional and psychological impact of mass casualty incidents on forensic odontologists. J Forensic Sci 2002;47(3):539–41.

[86] Pretty IA, Webb DA, Sweet D. The design and assessments of mock mass disasters for dental personnel. Journal of Forensic Sciences 2001;46(1):74–9.

ELSEVIER
SAUNDERS

Dent Clin N Am 51 (2007) 857–869

THE DENTAL CLINICS OF NORTH AMERICA

Pharmaceuticals and the Strategic National Stockpile Program

Amy Stewart, MPH[a,*], Geoffrey A. Cordell, PhD[b]

[a]*Division of Disaster Planning & Readiness, Illinois Department of Public Health, 500 E. Monroe Street, Springfield, IL 62701, USA*

[b]*Disaster Emergency Medicine Readiness Training Center, College of Dentistry, University of Illinois at Chicago, 801 S. Paulina Street, Chicago, IL 60612, USA*

In September and October 2001, two waves of attacks from anthrax (*Bacillus anthracis*) contained in mailed letters were conducted on the East Coast of the United States. Twenty-two people were infected with inhalation anthrax as a result, and of those 22, 5 died [1]. Two of the letters, which were apparently sent from a mail box in Princeton, NJ, were addressed to Senators Tom Daschle of South Dakota and Patrick Leahy of Vermont. Within one of the envelopes was a note with a pharmaceutical direction "Take Penacilin [sic] Now." The earlier group of five letters contained a brown granular form of anthrax and caused lesions of cutaneous anthrax. The other two letters contained approximately 1 g of more potent, white, refined anthrax spores that subsequently caused inhalation anthrax. Both samples originated from the same strain (Ames), and were derived from the original-type strain studied by the United States Army Medical Research Institute of Infectious Diseases at Fort Detrick, MD. The level of sophistication and technology to produce the second batch of anthrax spores is significant, but the laboratory that originated this material has yet to be found. Despite more than 9000 interviews on six continents, no one has been held responsible. It is estimated that more than $1 billion was spent on providing prophylactic medications and clean-up operations at various federal locations as a result of the attacks [1].

This was not the first attack on the United States using a biologic weapon. A significant number (at least 239) of mock "attacks" took place in the late 1940s and into the 1960s as the US government live-tested various

* Corresponding author.
E-mail address: amy.stewart@illinois.gov (A. Stewart).

0011-8532/07/$ - see front matter
doi:10.1016/j.cden.2007.06.001

bacteria over San Francisco from a Navy ship and dropped biologic agents over New York, Washington, DC, and Panama City, FL to determine the spread of the particles and how easy it would be to conduct such an attack [2]. Until Senate hearings in 1977, these tests were not general public knowledge. One such attack—on the New York subway system in midtown Manhattan—involved dropping light bulbs filled with *Bacillus subtilis* var. *niger* on the train tracks. The Army report on the incident concluded, "Similar covert attacks with a pathogenic agent during peak traffic periods could be expected to expose large numbers of people to infection and subsequent illness or death" [2].

Biologic warfare, in the form of clay pots filled with rotting "serpents of every kind," was probably instigated by Hannibal as a key element of his victory over King Eumenes of Perganum in 184 BC. In the Middle Ages, the Tartars propelled plague-ridden bodies over the walls of Caffa to cause plague in the enemy, and similar tactics were used by the Russians against Sweden in 1710. Smallpox was used in the fifteenth and eighteenth centuries as a weapon through the distribution of contaminated clothing. For example, during the French and Indian wars, smallpox-laden blankets were supplied by the English to Native Americans. Similar incidents of biologic weapon use involving cholera and the plague also may have occurred during World War I in Italy and Russia, respectively [2]. Chemical weapons use (chlorine gas) was initiated in Ypres, Belgium by German forces in 1915.

In June 1925, the Protocol for the Prohibition of the Use in War of Asphyxiating, Poisonous or Other Gases and of Bacteriological Methods of Warfare was developed and is known as the Geneva Protocol [3,4]. Unfortunately, it contained no provision for monitoring and inspection regarding compliance. In 1932, the Japanese government began a substantial biologic weapons program that was subsequently inflicted on China and resulted in untold deaths from bubonic plague. In 1940, on Gruinard Island in Scotland, the British developed anthrax "bombs" that demonstrated effectiveness against sheep. At the conclusion of the tests, the island was so dangerous that it remained off limits (and classified) until decontaminated with formaldehyde in 1986. Subsequently, anthrax was described as being "100-1000 times more potent than any chemical agent" [1].

It was in 1953 that research was initiated in the United States on the defensive aspects of biologic weapons, including vaccines, chemoprophylaxes, and therapeutic regimens. Subsequently, in 1969, President Richard Nixon signed an executive order that the US offensive program would be terminated and only small research quantities of biologic agents would be retained for the development of biologic protective measures, diagnostic procedures, and therapeutic regimens. The 1972 Biological Weapons Convention (implemented in 1975) was signed by 140 countries and was supposed to halt the proliferation of biologic agents and eliminate current offensive weapon stockpiles. The use of such agents in "defensive" research was not subject to direct oversight. Based on an incident of inhalation anthrax, in which 66 people died in Sverdlovsk, Russia in April 1979, it became clear (from President Yeltsin in 1992) that the Soviet Union had at least one secret biologic warfare facility. In actuality, the program had more than 40 such facilities and at its peak employed more than 50,000 scientists and technicians. The dispersal of these scientific personnel and their associated knowledge and materiel after the 1989 dissolution of the Soviet Union is of grave and continuing concern [2]. The Japanese religious cult Aum Shinrikyo, which attacked the Tokyo subway with sarin gas in March 1995 and killed 12 people, also had a biologic weapons program and was attempting to develop *B anthracis*, *Clostridium botulinum*, and *Coxiella burentii* in weaponized forms [5]. A chemical weapons convention was signed in 1993 to provide a comprehensive ban on the development, production, stockpiling, and use of chemical weapons with guidelines for destruction of existing weapons. It came into force in 1997.

Vulnerability

The assessment of threat has been described as being a combination of the "perceived adversary's capability to produce and effectively disseminate biological agents, his intent to do so, and our own vulnerability to such an action" [2]. In practice, however, we can only assess our own vulnerabilities. The focus at federal and local levels is on using our existing and emerging technologies to develop preventive and therapeutic measures for deployment. At the same time, we know that recombinant DNA techniques could produce modified organisms against which no preventive and therapeutic strategy could be developed. These organisms and known lethal strains of existing organisms and synthetic and natural chemical agents are regarded as "asymmetric threats." They represent weapons for which developing strategies to detect and respond to them to protect public health is substantially more difficult, particularly in the hands of terrorist groups that do not represent a particular sovereign nation.

An underlying assumption in planning for chemical and biologic threats also focuses on people as the principal point of attack. In reality, biologic and chemical attacks easily could be directed toward crops (eg, the use of Agent Orange in the Vietnam War), food animals, or biologically degradable plastics and rubber. In considering the use of available natural, chemical, and biologic toxins, a plethora of such agents is beyond the classic agents that cause anthrax, smallpox, or the plague. The Centers for Disease Control and Prevention's (CDC) list of critical biological agents (categories A, B, and C) does not include many of these agents because they are viewed as not being capable of development as threats.

From a response-planning perspective, what is the potential local impact of such an attack? A 1997 study published by the CDC estimated that an attack with *B anthracis* on a town of 100,000 people would result in 50,000 cases of illness and 32,875 deaths [6]. Only through environmental surveillance and the early administration of appropriate antibiotics could such a disaster of mortality be modulated. Any act of terrorism (or a large-scale natural disaster) targeting the US civilian population will require rapid access to large quantities of pharmaceutical agents and medical supplies. Such quantities of medication and medical supplies may not be readily available locally, and quantities available will be depleted quickly. Preparedness for biologic or chemical attack and natural disasters requires consideration of the accumulation (stockpiling) of adequate pharmaceutical and associated medical supplies.

History of federal government pharmaceutical response

The first federally mandated stockpiles were overseen by the CDC, which is 1 of 13 major operating components of the Department of Health and Human Services. From 1974 until 1998, the primary focus of these programs was on naturally occurring infectious diseases, such as smallpox.

The Aum Shinrikyo sarin attack in 1995 raised legitimate concerns as to how a major city in the United States would respond pharmaceutically to such an attack from a chemical or biologic agent. In addition to the known cultivation of biologic agents by Aum Shinrikyo, intelligence exists to support that Iran, Syria, Libya, China, North Korea, Russia, Israel, Taiwan, and possibly Sudan, India, Pakistan, and Kazakhstan support offensive biologic weapons programs [2]. As a result, in 1999, the US Congress mandated the formation of the national pharmaceutical stockpile program. The program was appropriated $51 million to acquire and oversee the stockpile of pharmaceutical interventions, medical supplies, and equipment for immediate availability to a state or local authority making a request [7]. In March 2003, the national pharmaceutical stockpile program was shifted under the auspices of the US Department of Homeland Security and was renamed the Strategic National Stockpile (SNS) program [8]. With the signing of the BioShield legislation, the SNS program was returned to US Department of Health and Human Services for oversight and guidance.

Current stockpiling practices

The SNS program works with governmental and nongovernmental partners to upgrade the nation's public health capacity to respond to a national emergency. Critical to the success of this initiative is ensuring that capacity is developed at federal, state, and local levels to receive, stage, distribute, and dispense SNS assets. SNS past responses include the World Trade Center response on September 11, 2001, the anthrax response in October 2001, and the Hurricane Katrina and Rita responses in August and September 2005.

Strategic National Stockpile deployment

The goal of SNS is to transport a first wave of critically needed supplies to a requesting state within hours of the federal decision to deploy [8]. The deployed materiel may consist of a 12-hour push package, vendor-managed inventory, or other various needed medical materials. After the initial push package deployment, event-specific shipments are organized and released to state and local agencies in need.

The 12-hour push package

Twelve-hour push packages strategically located throughout the United States provide a broad-spectrum support that enables assets to be received within 12 hours after a federal decision has been made, and it will be deployed. Each push package is composed of large quantities of pharmaceutical agents, equipment, and medical supplies to begin individual 10-day regimens for more than 300,000 people. The push package is composed of more than 100 containers and weighs approximately 50 tons. It is designed to be transported either via cargo plane or trailer unit and requires more than 12,000 sq ft of space at the receiving site for full implementation. Because the package is preassembled before an event, the supplies are broad in scope. Each package contains unit dose and bulk oral antibiotics, oral antibiotic suspensions and syrups, intravenous and intramuscular injection medications, a selection of analgesic agents, and other emergency medications. There is equipment to be used in a mass-casualty event for tablet counting, volume counting, and automated packaging and medical supplies for intravenous administration and trauma care [8]. Push packages do not contain antitoxins and vaccines for category A biologic threat agents, such as anthrax, botulism, plague, smallpox, and tularemia. The SNS maintains separate stockpiles of these interventions and provides them in a separate shipment within the same time frame.

In support of the push package there is a five- to seven-person Technical Advisory Response Unit that deploys—ideally before the push package arrives at the site—to assist state and local authorities in receiving, managing, distributing, dispensing, and replenishing the push package. The unit also assists in providing packaging expertise and postevent recovery of assets to the push package site of origin. States are responsible for the development of their own plans for managing and distributing these assets and organizing teams of health care professionals to use them [8].

Managed inventory

Managed inventory is composed of federally owned inventory at vendor sites that can be deployed when needed as a follow-up to a push package or when an event is not large enough to justify a full 12-hour push package. Managed inventory is used to provide needed medications, as was evidenced after Hurricane Katrina, when badly needed medications were used for chronically ill patients. These supplies are tailored to the specific event and are intended for delivery within 12 hours or less when intended as a replacement for a push package or within 24 to 36 hours when intended as a secondary asset [8].

Federal Medical Station

A newly developed SNS asset that was deployed for the first time after Hurricane Katrina is the Federal Medical Station (FMS) [9]. The FMS is a medical asset that is designed to support regional, state, and local health care agencies that respond to catastrophic events that have damaged, incapacitated, or overwhelmed existing medical facilities. The basic type III FMS is a low- to mid-acuity of care and has supplies and pharmaceutical agents to treat approximately 250 people for approximately 3 days. The asset provides the following critical capabilities: (1) inpatient, nonacute treatment capability for areas in which hospital bed capacity has been exceeded, (2) a special needs shelter for displaced persons with chronic diseases, limited mobility, or behavioral health requirements, and (3) support to quarantine missions that isolate persons suspected of being exposed to or affected by a highly contagious disease. Type I FMSs are for critical care settings and Type II FMSs are specialized critical care units. The FMS provides shelter and medical supplies; however, a professional staff is required to implement and augment the station [9]. A local team of trained medical professionals, such as dentists and dental hygienists, would be an important adjunct to assist with the FMS deployment on site.

Local stockpiling challenges

Although SNS is designed to support state and local response efforts, it is not intended to replace or supplant local preparedness efforts. Planned delivery of a push package is within 12 hours of the federal decision to deploy, however. The SNS does not supply personnel or explicit instructions for dispensation, so the task of distribution and patient prioritization for treatment and prophylaxis remains the responsibility of state and local planning agencies. After the attacks on September 11, 2001 and the anthrax attacks shortly thereafter, Havlak and coworkers [10] at the CDC indicated 11 challenges extant with the creation of a pharmaceutical stockpile designed to respond to a terrorist event (Box 1).

These challenges are mostly logistical and managerial, and the authors describe some of the steps taken by the CDC to ameliorate them. The actual materiel supplied through the (then) national pharmaceutical stockpile (currently SNS) does not seem to have been regarded as a challenge and illustrates the federal government's focus on national distribution rather than community planning. The inability of pharmaceutical supply to keep pace with demand and the nonexistence of pharmaceutical interventions for particular agents (eg, viral hemorrhagic fevers) was not addressed. Three community-specific challenges associated with the stockpiling requirement are financial burden, coordinating personnel to implement distribution and dispensing plans, and materiel selection.

Box 1. Challenges to creating a pharmaceutical stockpile

Political support
Fiscal support
Centralized versus decentralized stockpiles
Stockpile organization
Stockpile oversight
Determining a procurement partner
Determining a product management partner
Determining storage sites
Determining transport partners
Preparing unit dose prophylactic regimens
Ensuring effective management and use in a deployment

How additional antibiotics, other therapeutic agents, and medical supplies are stockpiled and distributed remains a critical and controversial issue; the cost of establishing and maintaining a local stockpile places strain on tight budgets, so the selection of appropriate interventions in appropriate amounts is critical. There is no national consensus on what constitutes an adequate stockpile, which makes long-term budget strategies difficult [11]. This is illustrated by the undersupply and static stockpile inventory. The cost-benefit for local inventory enhancement is related to the probability of an attack. For smaller communities, there is a relatively high initial inventory cost, followed by the ongoing replacement costs to maintain contemporary stocks, which these communities may be unable to afford. This cost, coupled with the low probability of attack, decreases the overall benefit of the stockpile to the small community [12]. Hsu and coworkers [13] of Johns Hopkins University in Baltimore have questioned whether regional hospital pharmacies are prepared for public health emergencies. They conducted a survey of 22 acute care hospitals in the Maryland region and found that of the 19 respondents, 74% had reserve pharmaceutical supplies for chemical and biologic events and 58% had supplies for radiologic events. For the six CDC category A biologic threats (anthrax, plague, and tularemia), ciprofloxacin and doxycycline are recommended and were key pharmaceuticals assessed in the stockpiling. It was calculated that there would be a need for 863,112 oral doses required for these two drugs in the hospitals surveyed, given the population distribution. Only 286,464 oral doses were available for prophylaxis, however, and only 2698 intravenous doses were available for treatment, compared with a likely need for 13,200 doses. Only 446 regional doses of the two drugs for pediatric use were reported.

Adequate pharmaceutical support for this segment of the population remains a challenge. A suggestion was made from the hospitals surveyed that a regional pharmaceutical stockpile was needed [13]. A recent study conducted in Los Angeles County of 45 hospitals focused more on overall preparedness and barely touched on pharmaceutical stockpiling as an important factor [14]. Half of the hospitals had a chemical antidote stockpile, and 42% had an antibiotic stockpile (specific agents not disclosed). An earlier survey examined the effects of the Weapons of Mass Destruction Act of 1996 and particularly compared the levels of chemical antidote stocks available in one US city [15]. At the time of the survey in July 2000 there was no difference in preparedness levels for nerve agent and cyanide antidotes from the July 1996 survey.

Regardless of stockpile size or contents, local communities are required to provide manpower and distribution; the largest, most comprehensive stockpile is useless if not distributed during an event. There is uncertainty regarding the capacity that individual communities should have for inventory distribution and dispensation [12]. The capability of a city to provide oral antibiotics within a 48-hour period after an event remains an important benchmark for local community plans, and yet evidence-based research on effective methods remains elusive [12]. To address some of these concerns, Baravata and coworkers [12] examined how mortality could be reduced from an anthrax bioterrorism attack through different strategic stockpiling and dispensing models. Importantly, they discovered that mortality depended critically on local dispensing capacity: Low distribution capacity leads to high mortality because of lack of treatment; high distribution capacity (14,000 per hour or more) leads to mortality because of lack of pharmaceutical regimen compliance. Finally, early event detection has a minimal effect on mortality in communities in which dispensing capacity is low; agent detection is most useful when response mechanisms meet the community needs created by instructions to seek medical care. To maximize community benefit, local priorities should focus on (1) maximizing local dispensing capacity, (2) encouraging education regarding prophylaxis or treatment regimens, and (3) introducing environmental sensing and detection technologies only after dispensing levels had been increased [12].

Several states have conducted exercises that involved evaluating the effectiveness of dispensing from the SNS [16–18]. An Iowa pharmacist group found that for a response to a statewide event, 300 dispensing sites involving up to eight pharmacists at each site would be needed. No mention was made of whether other health professionals familiar with certain types of drugs, such as dentists, could assist in the dispensing operations. Washington State also conducted an exercise in January 2002 that simulated a mass exposure to *B anthracis* with 230 volunteer patients, and the results of the patient and practitioner volunteer surveys were published [17,18]. One of the critical lessons learned was the importance of prior training so that workers would feel competent to respond under stress. In the last 2 years, local health departments and hospitals in Illinois have conducted exercises to test their ability to dispense medications within the 48-hour time frame as suggested by the CDC. Although several departments in the state proved that they could meet this task, many departments suggested that additional staff was needed to accomplish this task or alternate modalities needed to be considered. The Illinois Medical Response Team was developed in 1999 to respond to major incidents in which medical staffing may require augmentation. The group realized that the state as a whole needed a network of coordinated mutual support and a more systematic approach to responding to a large-scale catastrophe. Depending on the event, the Illinois Medical Response Team and other health care professionals associated with a medical facility may not be readily available to assist local agencies with mass dispensing or vaccination efforts, which reaffirms the need for preidentified medical volunteers who could be trained to assist with mass dispensing/vaccinations.

Cohen [19] discussed the development of a pharmacy emergency response team at the Maimonides Medical Center in Brooklyn, New York, after the events of 2001 discussed earlier. The professionals delineated as important for the team were pharmacy administrator, drug information pharmacist, intensive care unit pharmacist, infectious diseases pharmacist, nuclear pharmacist, management information system pharmacist, hazardous materials pharmacist, and auxiliary site pharmacist. The functions of the pharmacy emergency response team and its pharmaceutical care and operations management role as a part of an overall comprehensive response effort are described. In an interesting appendix, a formulary of stockpiled pharmaceutical agents is described for the treatment of up to 100 patients and the prophylactic use by 4000 persons after biologic, chemical, or radiologic attack [19].

Once a stockpile is established, its contents must be continually reassessed to maintain preparedness against emerging infectious diseases or new bioweapon threats. For example, according to the World Health Organization, avian influenza A (H5N1) has so far led to the deaths of 164 humans from a total of 256 cases in ten countries, mostly in Southeast Asia as of January 29, 2007. It first was noted as being lethal to humans through infected poultry in 1997 in Hong Kong, and because of its high lethality rate after infection, "bird flu" became a major news story globally in 2004 and 2005. There is a danger that mutation of the organism could occur and result in an orally transmissible strain (similar to tuberculosis). The World Health Organization considers the current alert for a pandemic to be at stage 3, indicating limited person-to-person transmission [20]. Serious preparations for antiviral stockpiling and enhanced vaccine production only recently have been initiated. Four antiviral agents currently on the market—amantadine (Symmetrel), rimantadine (Flumadine), zanamivir (Relenza), and oseltamivir (Tamiflu)—have been actively considered for local stockpiles. All four have some therapeutic and prophylactic efficacy; however, there is evidence of antiviral drug resistance to amantidine and rimantadine in strains in Thailand, Vietnam, and Cambodia [21–23]. The CDC, National Institutes of Health, and the US Food and Drug Administration added an 80% Tamiflu/20% Relenza allocation to the federal stockpile. The allocation was determined because of Tamiflu's ease of storage and administration; however, Tamiflu has a higher possibility of drug resistance. Relenza has a lower possibility of drug resistance but includes a black box warning for contraindication with chronic lung disease ailment because of risk of bronchospasms for these compromised individuals and difficulty in administering. For the purposes of the SNS assets, it was concluded that it was desirable to have some of both drugs. Vaccines are in the early stages of development but will not be fully refined until a particular strain emerges and therefore cannot be stockpiled.

For every addition to a stockpile inventory, public health agencies and community stakeholders must come together, weigh costs and benefits of inclusion, select an intervention among a pool of similar products, and assess the ability to acquire the selected product. Once product selection has occurred and acquisitions have begun, agencies must begin planning for the instance that adequate product is not available to meet community needs and establish patient priority policy.

Role of the dentist

At the time of a disaster, whether natural or man made, additional medical professionals are needed to distribute the medical supplies brought to the affected areas. In the case of an airborne anthrax event, the CDC's recommendation is to dispense antibiotic medications to the entire population within 48 hours. The responsibility of this task would fall to the public health sector and the medical providers in the community. Federal assets, such as the medication cache, would be delivered to the affected state(s) or area. State and local agencies work together to provide medications to the affected populations. Traditionally, public health is population-based health care; however, many public health agencies would not have the manpower to dispense medications or administer vaccines to the entire population within a 48-hour time period. In Illinois, the governing body of a local health department is the Board of Health, with a physician as the medical director. Many local health departments do not employ physicians as staff, however, because they do not provide direct patient care. In developing their emergency preparedness plans, public health agencies are looking to allied health professionals to assist with the task of dispensing medications within the first 48 hours.

In a national or state disaster, physicians affiliated with hospitals are tasked with the emergency at hand, making them unavailable for field or alternative care facility response. For example, if the SNS deployed a field medical station as a supplement to a local hospital, doctors from the local hospital should not be expected to man both facilities. Medical professionals who could provide additional assistance with mass dispensing or mass immunizations include—but would not be limited to—dentists, pharmacists, nurses, and veterinarians. Unlike pharmacists and nurses, dentists can administer and dispense medications, which makes them vital partners in a mass clinic. Other functions at a mass clinic with which dentists could assist include triage, screening patients, and care of patients who present at the clinic. In an emergency, alternate treatment sites and special needs shelters may be established to care for individuals who have suffered an exposure but are asymptomatic and populations that express a specific need or require special care. Dental professionals also could offer assistance at these various sites.

In June 2002, the American Dental Association held a meeting in an effort to identify the role of dentists in responding to a bioterrorism attack. By the conclusion of the meeting, the participants had identified several areas in which the dental profession may be called on to assist in the event of a major attack, including surveillance and notification, diagnosis and monitoring, referral, immunizations, medications, triage, medical care augmentation, decontamination, and infection control. In preparation for dentists to play a role in an emergency, it was determined that incorporating bioterrorism training into the existing dental curriculum could be implemented easily [24]. Dental professionals could fill a various roles, ranging from clerical to inventory management, in a mass clinic, shelter, or alternate treatment site.

In the last 2 years, much progress has been made in changing laws to increase the workforce of medical professionals in an emergency. With the passing of the Illinois Emergency Powers Act, the scope of practice for licensed professionals may be modified if certain criteria are met. Effective January 1, 2006, Illinois Public Act 94-409 added the definition of a dental emergency responder, which could provide medical care within the scope of practice of any dentist or dental hygienist who is certified in emergency medical response during a declared local, state, or national emergency.

Preidentification and specific training of emergency workers before an actual event can save critical minutes when the event does occur. Medical volunteers also have been identified as public health first responders and are included with other responders when emergency supplies and medications are distributed. Local agencies at the city or county level are the focal point of emergency planning efforts because they are in the best position to coordinate with the county offices of emergency management and other public and private organizations in the area. In Illinois, city and county public health departments have been working with medical reserve corps, community providers, and county emergency management agencies to develop a medical volunteer base to assist public health in an emergency. The collaboration of agencies and individuals organizing together will strengthen the infrastructure so that they can respond effectively should a disaster occur.

Summary

Preparedness activities that began before September 11, 2001 have been expanded, and new programs have resulted from federal, state, and local policies toward an all-hazards approach. The all-hazards approach will prepare a community better for any emergency, whether natural or man made. If a large-scale emergency hits, communities must look within their own resources to provide assistance in the first few hours. Trained volunteers, such as dental professionals, are a much needed resource to assist physicians and other medical professionals in the time of need.

When asked, "Are we prepared?" Dr. Julie Gerberding, Director of the CDC, responded, "The answer is that it is the wrong question. Preparedness is not a black-or-white event. It is an ongoing process of improvement" [25]. The continued support and involvement of the dental community, in collaboration with the medical community, will provide one facet of the improvement necessary for an effective response effort.

References

[1] Canter DA. Remediating anthrax-contaminated sites: learning from the past to protect the future. Chemical Health & Safety 2005;12:13–9.

[2] Noah DL, Huebner KD, Darling RG, et al. The history and threat of biological warfare and terrorism. Emerg Med Clin North Am 2002;20:255–71.

[3] Geissler E, editor. Biological and toxin weapons today. Oxford (England): Oxford University Press; 1986.

[4] Available at: http://en.wikipedia.org/wiki/Geneva_Protocol. Accessed February 2, 2007.

[5] Sidell FR, Franz DR, editors. Medical aspects of chemical and biological warfare. Washington, DC: Borden Institute; 1997. p. 1–7.

[6] Kaufmann AF, Meltzer MI, Schmid GP. Emerg Infect Dis 1997;3:83–94.

[7] Combating terrorism: chemical and biological medical supplies are poorly managed. GAO/HEHS/AIMD-00-36. Washington, DC: Government Accounting Office; 1999. p. 26.

[8] Esbitt D. The strategic national stockpile: roles and responsibilities of health care professionals for receiving stockpile assets. Disaster Manag Resp 2003;1:68–70.

[9] Available at: http://www.texasjrac.org/documents/fmsfactsheet3–1.pdf. Accessed February 5, 2007.

[10] Havlak R, Gorman SE, Adams SA. Challenges associated with creating a pharmaceutical stockpile to respond to a terrorist event. Clin Microbiol Infect 2006;8:529–33.

[11] Terriff CM, Tee AM. Citywide pharmaceutical preparation for bioterrorism. Am J Health Syst Pharm 2001;58:233–7.

[12] Bravata DM, Zaric GS, Holty J-EC, et al. Reducing mortality from anthrax bioterrorism: strategies for stockpiling and dispensing medical and pharmaceutical supplies. Biosecur Bioterror: Biodef Strat Prac Sci 2006;4:244–62.

[13] Hsu EB, Casani JA, Roamnosky A, et al. Are regional hospital pharmacies prepared for public health emergencies? Biosecur Bioterror: Biodef Strat Prac Sci 2006;4:237–43.

[14] Kaji AH, Lewis RJ. Hospital disaster preparedness in Los Angeles County. Acad Emerg Med 2006;13:1198–203.

[15] Keim ME, Pesik N, Twum-Danso NA. Lack of hospital preparedness for chemical terrorism in a major US city: 1996–2000. Prehospital Disaster Med 2003;18:193–9.

[16] Young D. Iowa pharmacists dispense from strategic national stockpile during drill. Am J Health Syst Pharm 2003;60:1304–5.

[17] Beaton RD, Oberle MW, Wicklund J, et al. Evaluation of the Washington State National Pharmaceutical Stockpile dispensing exercise: Part I. Patient volunteer findings. J Public Health Manag Pract 2003;9:368–76.

[18] Beaton RD, Stevermer A, Wicklund J, et al. Evaluation of the Washington State National Pharmaceutical Stockpile dispensing exercise: Part II. Dispensary site worker findings. J Public Health Manag Pract 2004;10:77–85.

[19] Cohen V. Organization of a health-system pharmacy team to respond to episodes of terrorism. Am J Health Syst Pharm 2003;60:1257–63.
[20] Juckett G. Avian influenza: preparing for a pandemic. Am Fam Physician 2006;74:783–90.
[21] Ward P, Small I, Smith J, et al. Oseltamivir (Tamiflu) and its potential for use in the event of an influenza pandemic. J Antimicrob Chemother 2005;(55 Suppl S1):i5–21.
[22] Hayden FG. Antivirals for pandemic influenza. J Infect Dis 1997;(176 Suppl 1):S56–61.
[23] Hayden FG. Pandemic influenza: is an antiviral response realistic? Pediatr Infect Dis J 2004; 23:S262–9.
[24] Chmar JE, Ranney RR, Guay AH, et al. Incorporating bioterrorism training into dental education: report of ADA-ADEA terrorism and mass casualty curriculum development workshop. J Dent Educ 2004;68(11):1196–8.
[25] Ziskin LZ, Burke MV. New Jersey State program development for terrorism preparedness and other public health emergencies. N J Med 2004;101(9):17.

ELSEVIER
SAUNDERS

THE DENTAL CLINICS OF NORTH AMERICA

Dent Clin N Am 51 (2007) 871–878

Engaging the Dental Workforce in Disaster Mitigation to Improve Recovery and Response

Nicholas G. Mosca, DDS[a,b,*]

[a]*Division of Health Services, Mississippi State Department of Health, 570 East Woodrow Wilson Street, Jackson, MS 39215-1700, USA*
[b]*Department of Pediatric and Public Health Dentistry, University of Mississippi School of Dentistry, 2500 North State Street, Jackson, MS 39216, USA*

Background and significance

> "Natural hazards are a part of life. But hazards only become disasters when people's lives and livelihoods are swept away...let us remind ourselves that we can and must reduce the impact of disasters by building sustainable communities that have long-term capacity to live with risk."
> —Kofi Annan, Secretary-General of the United Nations, on the occasion of the International Day for Disaster Reduction, October 8, 2003.

The aftermath of Hurricane Katrina spotlighted many far-reaching consequences beyond the local loss of lives and properties, including the displacement of more than 750,000 victims, an increase in global fuel prices after the closure of oilrigs in the Gulf of Mexico, and even a record trade deficit for the United Kingdom [1]. Hurricane Katrina affected the lives and the livelihoods of many health professionals, and the destruction of public health and medical care infrastructure in the affected areas was unprecedented. All 14 hospitals and three federal medical facilities in the lower six counties of Mississippi were damaged, and 11 hospitals in the New Orleans area were flood-bound. Sanders [2] reported that Louisiana State University Health Sciences Center's School of Medicine experienced a significant loss in patients, departmental faculty and staff, practice and office space, and graduate medical education funding and subsequently

* Mississippi State Department of Health, 570 East Woodrow Wilson Street, Jackson, MS 39215-1700.
E-mail address: nicholas.mosca@msdh.state.ms.us

doi:10.1016/j.cden.2007.06.005 *dental.theclinics.com*

lost millions of dollars in clinic revenue. The impact on health care systems was also far-reaching. The University of Texas MD Anderson Cancer Center reported having operational losses of $16 million caused by a loss of hotel beds for their consultation patients, loss of referring physicians, and a 4-day operations shutdown in response to Hurricane Rita in September 2005 [3].

Sariego [4] observed that disasters create chaos and disrupt the normal functioning of the affected community, including its health care infrastructure and resources. Many publications in the aftermath of Hurricane Katrina described how a lack of hospitals and physicians impacted the delivery of medical services, but they largely ignored how the disaster affected the delivery of nonallopathic services, such as dental care. The American Dental Association reported that Hurricane Katrina affected the lives of an estimated 1185 licensed dentists, 49% of whom lived in Louisiana and 21% in Mississippi [5]. In September 2005, an initial assessment of the affected areas in Mississippi revealed that more than 85 dental offices were partially or completely destroyed and 44 dentists lost their homes.

Estimating that the average dentist provides care to 52.2 patients per week, more than 303,000 monthly patient visits were disrupted in the immediate recovery after the storm, which resulted in an estimated revenue loss of $63 million per month [5]. Subsequently, many dentists experienced prolonged displacement and family disruptions, some experienced the complete loss of their business, and some experienced the loss of patients and auxiliary staff, which motivated some dental workers to consider relocation from the affected areas to avoid financial hardships. Individuals who experienced Hurricane Katrina have a better understanding of disaster preparedness through the hardships endured and the lessons learned. The dental profession, by virtue of its commitment to comprehensive primary health care, should be as engaged as allopathic providers in disaster mitigation planning. By participating in emergency management planning, the dental profession can mitigate prolonged recovery of the dental care infrastructure and improve the odds of having sustainable systems of dental care in the aftermath of devastation.

Mitigation is the process of anticipating risks to life and property and implementing actions that reduce or eliminate these risks. It is the first phase of emergency management planning that also includes preparedness, response, and recovery in the national response plan [6]. Mitigation is used to implement long-term measures to prevent hazards from developing into disasters altogether or reduce the effects of disasters (Fig. 1).

Effective mitigation planning identifies and evaluates hazards and makes predictions by measuring risks and vulnerability from such hazards. Mitigation may reduce or eliminate risk from hazards: the higher the risk, the more urgent the need to minimize hazards through mitigation. Structural mitigation uses technology-based measures (eg, construction of flood levees or installation of automatic shut-off valves for gas lines) to reduce or eliminate

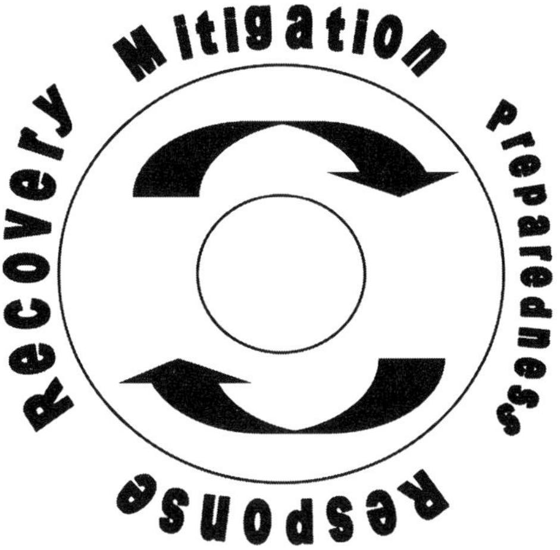

Fig. 1. Phases of emergency management planning. (*Adapted from* Federal National Response Plan, US Department of Homeland Security.)

damage. Nonstructural mitigation uses legislation, regulations, and insurance (eg, authorization of land-use zoning to turn flood-prone areas into nonresidential natural habitats) or insurers managing and underwriting hazard insurance.

The dental profession should use mitigation planning to anticipate the risk for hazards and determine where it is safe to build or purchase a clinic facility. Areas that have a higher risk of flooding can be identified by review of topographic flood plain maps to identify flood-prone areas. Dentists can plan by identifying the zoning and building code requirements at the proposed clinic site. The purchase of property that is exposed to flooding or coastal erosion of storm surge should be avoided; the dentist should consider relocating the property to higher ground or ensure that the facility is constructed on posts high above the flood plain. The Federal Emergency Management Agency (FEMA) provides access to flood plain maps that can be viewed online at the FEMA mitigation Web site (Fig. 2) at http://msc.fema.gov/webapp/wcs/stores/servlet/FemaWelcomeView?storeId=10001&catalogId=10001&langId=-1.

Dental providers may not have the knowledge or time required to effectively anticipate hazards and risks. Professional hazard mitigation specialists can be used to perform risk assessment surveys and make recommendations on the purchase of property or hazard-related insurance. Mitigation planning differs by geographic location and the probability of risks that occurs in that location. For example, mitigation planning in communities with greater risk for earthquake or high-strength winds may incorporate seismic design standards and wind-bracing requirements in building design and construction to mitigate risk. In the aftermath of a disaster, the federal

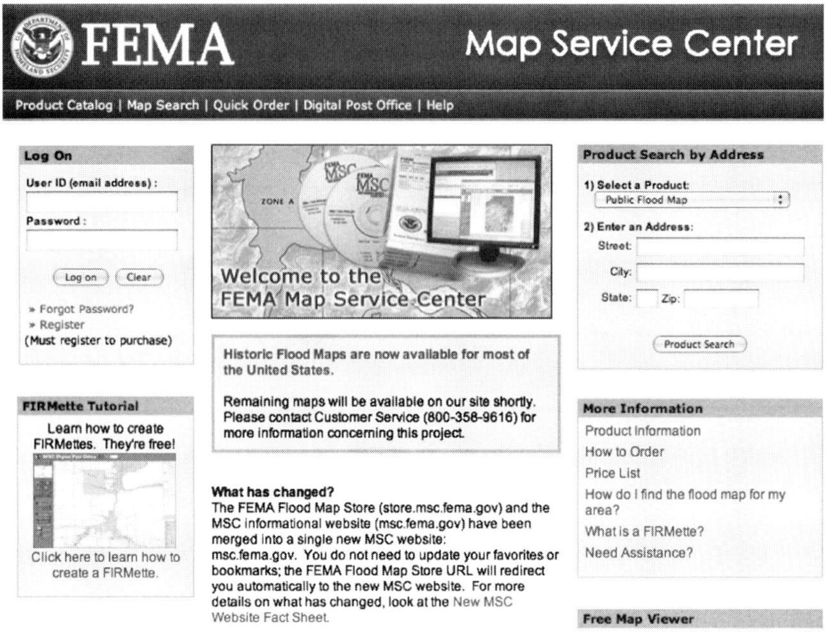

Fig. 2. FEMA mitigation Web site. (*From* Federal Emergency Management Agency. Available at: http://www.msc.fema.gov.)

government can provide mitigation support through Section 404 of the Robert T. Stafford Disaster Relief and Emergency Assistance Act. After a declaration of disaster has been made, FEMA is authorized to provide grants to states and local governments to implement long-term hazard mitigation measures. These grants may be used to elevate flood-prone structures, retrofit structures to minimize damage in future disasters, and make building code improvements during postdisaster reconstruction. FEMA provides information about the National Flood Insurance Program on the Web at http://www.fema.gov/about/programs/nfip/index.shtm and offers an online mitigation best practices portfolio at http://www.fema.gov/plan/prevent/bestpractices/index.shtm.

Comprehensive mitigation planning also should anticipate and prepare for the risks posed by environmental health effects and communicable disease outbreaks. An immediate consequence of natural disasters is the loss of water for drinking and handwashing, spoilage of food from the lack of refrigeration, and loss of functional sanitation facilities [7]. Environmental exposure to mercury, radiation, and organic compounds used in disinfection may occur as a result of the devastation of a dental clinic facility. The dental profession should advocate for additional state and federal resources to mitigate the environmental impact of these potential exposures. FEMA provides information about environmental contamination risks and has links to resources for natural disasters action plans on its Web site at http://www.epa.gov/greenkit/q5_disas.htm [8].

A personal mitigation plan for dentists, their families, and staff is recommended to anticipate the loss of basic resources such as water, electricity, gas, and telephones. Emergency preparedness kits can be assembled that contain essential supplies, including flashlights, fresh batteries, battery-powered radio, basic medical aid supplies, and nonperishable foods and drinking water to last several days. Reminder checklists of the important steps to take before, during, and after a disaster should be kept in a handy location because a disaster can strike quickly and without warning. A listing of local evacuation procedures should be included with the checklists. The location of emergency shelters and back-up suppliers for vital resources, such as gasoline and water, should be identified. Employees and family members should share contact information, including cell phone numbers, email addresses, and a location where they plan to stay during and after an emergency crisis event. Planning to ensure reliable modes of communication is essential. Hurricane Katrina's devastation revealed how all traditional modes of communication failed, including cell phone service. Text messaging proved to be the most reliable means of public communication in the affected areas.

Another consequence of devastation is the loss of staff and dental patients. In the aftermath of Hurricane Katrina, most providers did not anticipate the long-term dispersal of so many people across the nation. Many patients who remained locally in the aftermath of Hurricane Katrina were unable to contact their dental providers. Abdel-Monem and Bulling [9] noted an absence of understanding about the potential liability that mental health care providers face in the aftermath of disaster recovery. The potential liabilities that dental providers would face in Katrina's aftermath were unanticipated. For example, could dental patients claim abandonment because they were unable to contact their dental provider in a reasonable period of time after the disaster occurred? Dentists should prepare for the likely event that a dental practice will close for extended periods and inform patients about what to do if emergent care is needed and how treatment in progress will be completed (eg, the delivery of a denture).

Dentists can use mitigation planning to resume their clinical practice as quickly as possible by identifying an alternate location to temporarily relocate their dental practice in the event of building damage and having a plan to re-establish communication with patients. Important documents for clinical operations, such as verification of licensure, malpractice insurance, and patient records, should be stored in portable travel containers or copied and stored in a secure location for future retrieval. Providers can protect access to their patient records by using Web-accessible electronic patient records that allow the retrieval of databases from distant sites. Electronic dental records are widely available that include storage for digital photographs, which may assist with postmortem identification in mortuary operations. Databases should include patient contact information, including addresses of individuals' preferred evacuation sites, and all staff credentialing documentation, which ideally should be converted to digital format. If a cell phone number is recorded, it may be helpful to identify if the cell phone service allows text messaging. All patients should be informed of local hazard risks and receive guidance to prepare for disasters.

It is not an overstatement to say that the dental profession has a social responsibility to mitigate prolonged recovery of the dental care infrastructure and participate as health care providers in disaster response emergency services. Dentists should consider participation in local emergency response units. Local response units provide first response assistance to victims of disasters and coordinate early medical response. It is important to establish a sense of teamwork, strengthen communications for first responders, and understand the legal ramifications. Volunteer participants must receive emergency management training and education to participate. Many dentists have the capacity to perform various emergency response activities, including postmortem identification, assistance in fatality management, triage and prehospital care, and emergency dental treatment in mass care operations. Such social responsibility would provide community-level involvement and enhance long-term recovery. Dental education programs should prepare instruction and hands-on experiences for students and residents in all phases of emergency preparedness planning, including how traumatic events may affect them and their families emotionally to better prepare psychologically [10]. Students should receive instruction in the use of hazard mitigation maps to plan the location of a dental practice.

Most states have public health dental directors who provide leadership for state oral health programs in public health agencies. State oral health programs should participate in public health emergency planning and response at the state and local levels and be familiar with federal planning activities (Fig. 3). Readiness means the ability to respond immediately, and public health dental directors must know how best to act and cope during terrorism events and other public health emergencies. Dental directors should be familiar with emergency support function's #6, #8, and #14, the federal government's emergency response framework for mass care, public health and medical services, and community recovery and mitigation planning. Mississippi's experience in the aftermath of Hurricane Katrina demonstrated that the American public expects and demands efficient emergency public health and medical services. To improve these services, dentists must be included in multidisciplinary care response teams, and patient triage

National –	Resource Planning; Credentialing; National Stockpile Requests
State –	Sentinel Surveillance Planning; DMORT Planning; First Responder, Mass Care, & Triage Planning
Local –	Personal Preparedness Planning, Business Disaster Plan; Guidance for Patients

Fig. 3. Mitigation planning activities for state oral health programs.

and transfer operations should include access to emergency dental services [11].

State dental associations also should participate in clinical disaster planning activities. Comprehensive mitigation planning should include oral health services when determining what to do if victims are unable to access medications for several days and how to find future clinical care sites if an established clinic is nonfunctional (ie, Web addresses, toll-free telephone numbers). State oral health programs and state dental associations can participate collaboratively to identify how the scope and magnitude of social and economic disaster impacts the availability of urgent oral health care in the affected geographic region. In the aftermath of disaster, state oral health programs should be prepared to conduct rapid assessments to determine the impact on the dental care infrastructure and the loss of treatment resources. As a state health official, the public health dental director may initiate requests to obtain state or federal assistance for vital oral health resources once the declaration of emergency is issued. Incident-specific action requests can be submitted by the public health dental director to the state and federal government as part of the federal emergency support function's #8 interventions.

For effective response and recovery, public health dental directors should develop a disaster action plan to delineate specific agency participation to support specific community recovery and mitigation activities and cultivate alliances with other health programs located inside the region and outside the immediate area. A citywide or regional consortium of programs and hospitals may be able to assist in the rapid placement of mobile and portable equipment and trainees in the aftermath of the disaster [12]. The Emergency Management Assistance Compact, established in 1996, is a state-to-state compact that offers 50 states, the District of Columbia, Puerto Rico, and the US Virgin Islands the ability to share resources during a declaration of emergency. Emergency Management Assistance Compact agreements allows states to assist each other to identify available resources, negotiate reasonable resource costs, and deploy essential emergency and health workers through coordinated efforts. Emergency Management Assistance Compacts also address liability and credentialing issues within states. Action plans should include activities for postincident evaluation to measure the effectiveness of previous community recovery and mitigation efforts.

Summary

Dental professionals have a personal responsibility to ensure their dental staff's safety and a social responsibility to participate in mitigation planning to avoid prolonged recovery of the dental care infrastructure. Public health dental directors should work to convene federal, state, and local decision-making representatives to include the dental profession in emergency response planning to mitigate the impact of devastation on the primary oral health needs of individuals in the affected geographic areas. State dental associations should work with government agencies and emergency management groups to increase awareness of the importance for collaborative emergency response health services in the aftermath of natural disasters.

References

[1] McGuire WJ. Global risk from extreme geophysical events: threat identification and assessment. Philos Transact A Math Phys Eng Sci 2006;364(1845):1889–909.

[2] Sanders CV. Hurricane Katrina and the LSU-New Orleans department of medicine: impact and lessons learned. Am J Med Sci 2006;332(5):283–8.

[3] Konstanzer R, Colman G, Grisham JJ. Weathering a financial storm. Healthc Financ Manage 2006;60(9):50–4.

[4] Sariego J. A year after Hurricane Katrina: lessons learned at one coastal trauma center. Arch Surg 2007;142(2):203–5.

[5] Mississippi Dental Association and American Dental Association. Recovery empowerment summit: emerging from the storm. 2005. Conference Materials provided by the American Dental Association, 211 East Chicago Avenue, Chicago, IL 60611. Available at: http://www.dentrix.com/recovery%2Dempowerment%2Dsummit/. Accessed July 31, 2007.

[6] Federal Emergency Management Agency. National response plan. 2006. Available at: http://www.dhs.gov/xprepresp/committees/editorial_0566.shtm. Accessed April 6, 2007.

[7] Wilson JF. Health and the environment after Hurricane Katrina. Ann Intern Med 2006; 144(2):153–6.

[8] Natural Disasters Action Plan. US Environmental Protection Agency. Available at: http://www.epa.gov/greenkit/q5_disas.htm. Accessed April 13, 2007.

[9] Abdel-Monem T, Bulling D. Liability of professional and volunteer mental health practitioners in the wake of disaster: a framework for further consideration. Behav Sci Law 2005;23:573–90.

[10] More FG, Phelan J, Boylan R, et al. Predoctoral dental school curriculum for catastrophe preparedness. J Dent Educ 2004;68(8):851–8.

[11] Sariego J. Eight months later: Hurricane Katrina aftermath challenges facing the infectious diseases section of the Louisiana State University Health Science Center. Clin Infect Dis 2006;43(4):485–9 [E-pub 2006 Jul 5].

[12] Mosca NG, Finn E, Joskow R. Dental care as a vital service response for disaster victims. J Health Care Poor Underserved 2007;18(2):262–70.

ELSEVIER
SAUNDERS

THE DENTAL CLINICS OF NORTH AMERICA

Dent Clin N Am 51 (2007) 879–894

Oral Health Professionals Within State-Sponsored Medical Response Teams: The IMERT Perspective

Moses S. Lee, MD, FAAEM, FACEP[a,b,*], Bernard Heilicser, DO, MS, FACEP, FACOEP[c]

[a]*John H. Stroger Jr. Hospital of Cook County, Chicago, IL, USA*
[b]*Rush Medical University, Chicago, IL, USA*
[c]*Ingalls Memorial Hospital, Harvey, IL, USA*

There has always been a need for comprehensive, well-trained medical response teams in disaster events, including environmental catastrophes (eg, hurricanes, tornadoes, floods) and extreme heat and cold. Natural and man-made disasters, such as pandemic flu and industrial spills, respectively, can challenge our communities. They also include acts of terrorism, including chemical, biologic, radiologic, and nuclear warfare and explosives (CBRNE). Medical support during these times of domestic crises plays a significant role in the overall preparedness, response, and mitigation of such events. Federal teams have been well established in the form of disaster medical assistance teams (DMATs) [1]. A broad array of health care professionals has participated in DMATs, including dentists. Federal and local responses historically have formed a medical response in a disaster event. What has been lacking is an integrated state-based response team. In 1999, the State of Illinois recognized the need for a trained and credentialed medical response that can respond to any disaster within the state and bring health professionals, logistical support, supplies, and equipment to assist local providers when their resources are overwhelmed. With public health leadership, collaboration with nongovernmental agencies, and state public health allocation of federal funds, a volunteer team was created called the Illinois Medical Emergency Response Team (IMERT). This team included

* Corresponding author. Illinois Medical Emergency Response Team (IMERT), C/O Illinois College of Emergency Physicians, 1S280 Summit Ave., Court B-2, Oak Brook Terrace, IL 60181.
E-mail address: mlee@ccbh.org (M.S. Lee).

doi:10.1016/j.cden.2007.07.002 **dental.theclinics.com**

a broad array of individuals, including oral health care professionals, such as oral surgeons, dentists, and dental health hygienists. The following article reflects on the historical background of IMERT, its team development, partnerships, activations, and future directions with the integration of oral health care professionals as a vital resource for emergency response.

Historical background

Early in 1999, in response to the increased focus on terrorist threats and concern about deployment of weapons of mass destruction (WMD), a small group of emergency physicians, toxicologists, and emergency nurses began meeting with the Division of Emergency Medical Services of the Illinois Department of Public health (IDPH). Their initial intent was to assess the level of awareness and preparedness of emergency department personnel in Illinois to respond to a large-scale WMD incident. Such incidents would likely overwhelm public health agencies [2]. During this period, planning was underway to enhance emergency preparedness for a major incident in many large cities (eg, metropolitan medical strike teams) [3]. The Illinois group realized that the state needed a network of coordinated mutual support and a more systematic approach in the response to a large-scale catastrophe. The group realized that it was important to develop organized protocols, formalize communication systems, and recognize a core of specially prepared responders to assist in a case of mass casualty or WMD event. These responders also must be educated, trained, and cognizant of command systems.

In the summer of 1999, IDPH applied for and received a grant from the Centers for Disease Control and Prevention, which provided seed funding for IMERT. The funds were earmarked for the development of educational programs on emergency preparedness and the creation of infrastructure and equipment needed for medical response teams. Subsequent funding streams have been the Health Resources Services Administration, administered by IDPH, and Department of Homeland Security grants, administered by the Illinois Terrorism Task Force. The IMERT executive council was created to serve as oversight for IMERT. IMERT executive council members, who are emergency physicians, dentists, emergency nurses, and paramedics with extensive experience in emergency medical services (EMS) and disaster planning, are volunteers. They maintain leadership positions in their areas of employment. There are also selected individuals with military and technical expertise. The IMERT executive council has liaisons with advisors from IDPH, the Federal Bureau of Investigation, the US Public Health Services, and the Army Civil Support Team.

The mission of IMERT is to respond to and assist with emergency medical treatment at mass casualty incidents, including—but not limited to—environmental, chemical, biologic, and radiologic incidents, when activated by the director of IDPH or designee. IMERT is an integral part of the state medical disaster plan as depicted in the organizational chart (Fig. 1).

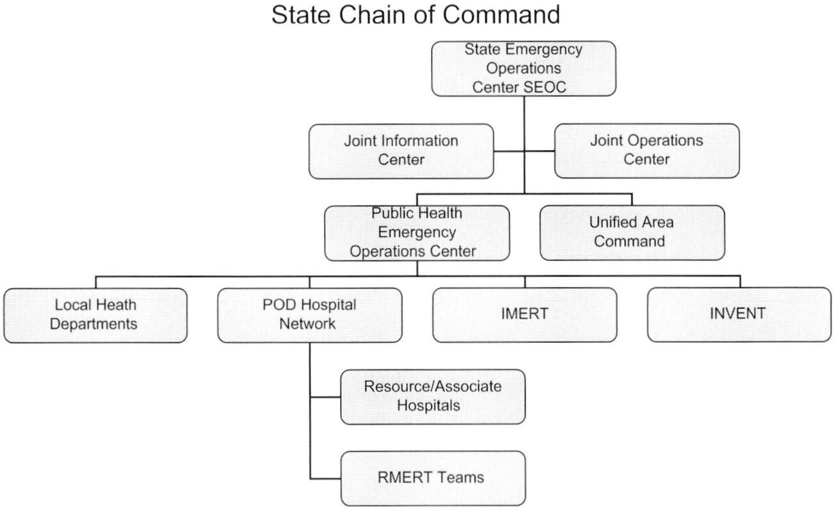

Fig. 1. Illinois medical disaster plan organizational chart.

Team development

The initial teams proposed consisted of a physician, nurse, an advanced life support specialist (EMT paramedic or intermediate), and a basic life support specialist (EMT-B). Their requirements were based on those advocated by federal DMATs but tailored toward the needs of the state. The requirements include online training composed of the National Incident Management System (NIMS), Federal Emergency Management Agency (FEMA) Incident Command System (ICS-100, -200), and a government-approved WMD course. Additional online training for administrators and training staff include the National Response Plan (NRP) IS-800 [4]. The team member applicant is also required to have current and unrestricted Illinois state licensure appropriate for his or her health care position. There is also a "boot camp" training session (Fig. 2). The first session was launched in June 2002. Boot camp is comprised of didactics on command structure, Illinois disaster medical response plan, equipment training, and various clinical skills workshops. Boot camp provides for team building and allows active members to participate in training sessions. In addition to online training and boot camp, the applicant also signs a "code of conduct" adapted from similar documents from federal teams and reviewed by a medical ethicist (coauthor Dr. B. Heilicser). Once members have completed requirements designated for their positions, they maintain their membership status by being on call for 2 weeks every 6 months and participation at least twice a year in drills or education activities or both. These extensive requirements ensure membership commitment and permit the various health care and non–health care volunteers to have the same baseline level of knowledge.

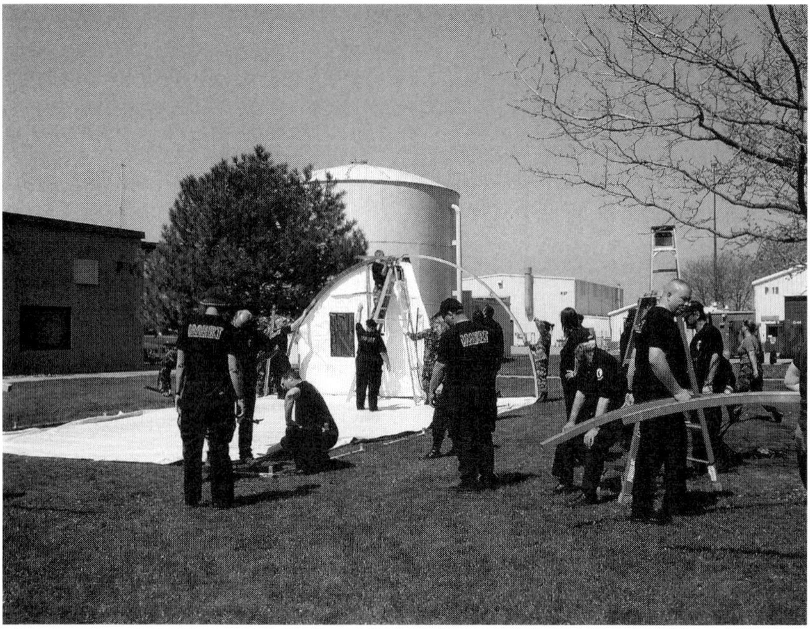

Fig. 2. IMERT boot camp activity (setting up medical care tents).

For example, a dental health care professional has experience with intraosseous insertions or learns to provide mass medical triage, items not typically presented in their daily practice. In addition to the inherent benefits of volunteer service to one's community, IMERT provides continuing education certificates for members based on their level of activity. These certificates can contribute to meeting a health care professional's state licensure requirements, including dentists.

The initial medical team has expanded significantly as more diverse individuals have expressed interest and IMERT has evolved and learned from each event, drill, or deployment. There are three types of teams: the general team, the state WMD team, and the urban search and rescue team. Overseeing these teams are command teams based on NIMS command structure with specific titles and duties. Knowledge of and compliance with NIMS allows IMERT to have parity with other agencies in terms of nomenclature and responsibilities. The command staff provides tactical and strategic support for the medical teams. Their main mission is to allow the medical teams to perform their duties in an efficient and productive fashion. The general teams have expanded their roster to include dentists and dental hygienists. Mental health professionals and pharmacists have been included. It also became evident that administrative support is critical in allowing practitioners to function properly. This acknowledgment led to the addition of safety, communication, logistical, and information technology specialists. There are two general teams on call at all times in each of the four regions in Illinois. The four regions are divided according to the Illinois Emergency Management Agency (IEMA) divisions (Fig. 3). IMERT responds within 4 hours of activation. IMERT may be tasked upon to mitigate an event or as an interim measure until the arrival of federal resources in a declared state of emergency. Federal support is extensive and massive, but it would

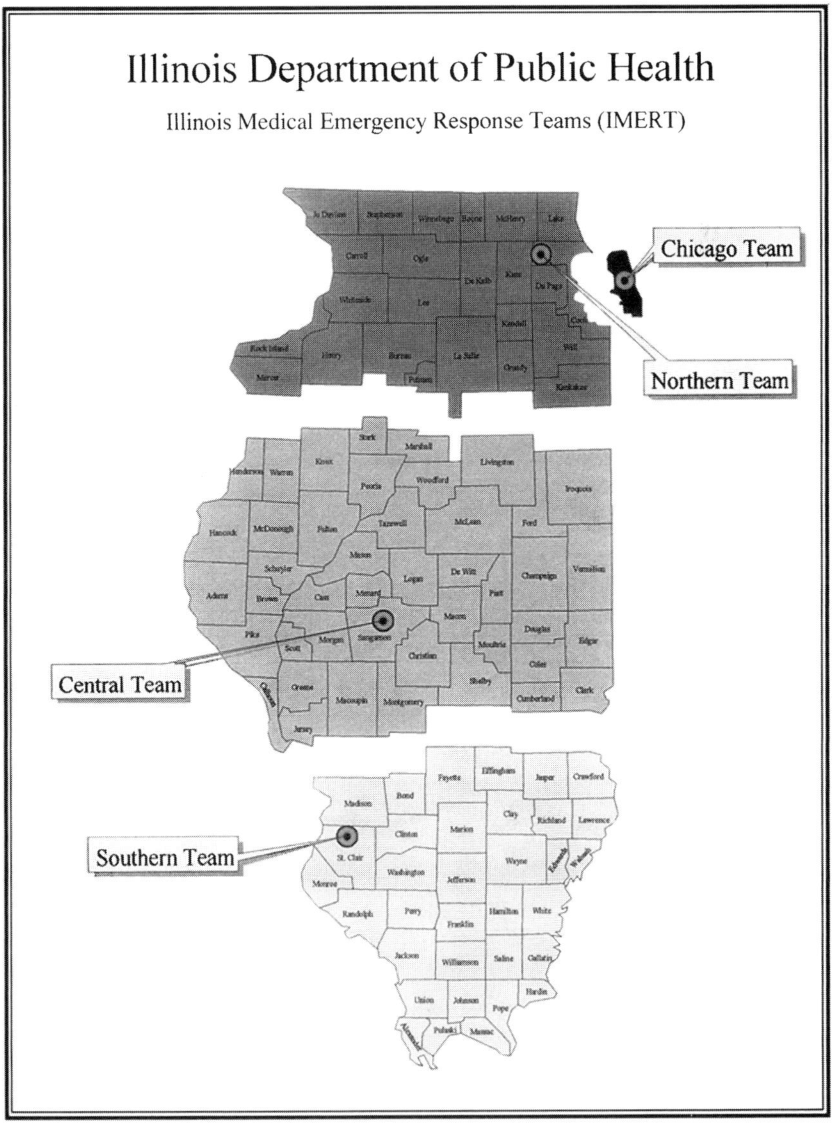

Fig. 3. IMERT regions.

take an average of 72 hours to mobilize [5]. IMERT members are given specific recommendations to be self-sufficient for at least 72 hours.

The IMERT state WMD team is the medical component of the Illinois state WMD. The Illinois state WMD team is a multiagency for the investigation and mitigation of a WMD incident. It consists of State of Illinois employees from the Illinois State Police, Illinois Environmental Protection Agency, IDPH, IEMA, and the Office of the State Fire Marshall [6]. The IMERT Urban Search and Rescue Team supplies the medical component to the Illinois Task Force 1 Urban Search and Rescue [7]. IMERT provides two medical teams on call at all times with these groups. Another group that germinated from IMERT is the Illinois Nurse Volunteer Emergency Needs Team (INVENT). They are activated to enhance an IMERT response and provide initial recovery phase health care.

This formalized approach to a medical response team provides collaborative opportunities for dentists and other oral health care professionals. In 2006, there were more than 9500 licensed dentists, and 80% were general dentists in Illinois [8]. Dentists have extensive knowledge of basic sciences and clinical skills and can be a valuable resource for emergency medical surge demands. A New York University Dental and Medical School 2002 survey of health professional leaders, including dental/medical school deans and dental/medical society presidents, showed a general agreement that dental professionals have an ethical obligation to assist during catastrophic events, but they also noted that they need disaster training and curriculum [9]. Dentists in the military have been shown to be capable of mass casualty triage [10]. Several publications have noted the potential role of dental professionals in emergency response [9,11–13]. A 2006 survey of dentists in Hawaii showed that only 2.3% of respondents reported having received prior bioterrorism preparedness training, and 14.5% felt that they were able to identify and recognize a bioterrorism event. A total of 73.8% indicated a willingness to provide assistance to the state in the event of a bioterrorism attack [13]. These findings lend support to the need for educational and training programs in order for dental health professionals to be properly prepared to assist a state. The dental community has much to offer in a disaster; they could assist in triage, medical evaluation and treatment, delivery of inoculations, providing analgesia, and health care administrative skills.

As the team composition evolved and grew, it became apparent that administrative and logistical supports are critical to optimal function of the medical teams. Their responsibilities include, but are not limited to, ensuring the safety of team members and the response site, maintaining adequate supplies, maintaining reliable lines of communications, providing information technology support, and ensuring reliability and safe transport of equipment. The primary goal of these team members is to guarantee the ability of the medical teams to deliver their services to the state of Illinois. Individual medical team members who have met the requirements for these roles have taken on logistical and administrative assignments, which provide another avenue of participation for oral health care professionals with additional nonclinical expertise.

The growth of the team in complexity and numbers requires a vast array of educational and training offerings. One advantage of a dental professional volunteering in IMERT is that the course requirements are also applicable to their daily work environment. For example, the NIMS curriculum from FEMA has been developed for responders. This common knowledge base allows responders from different jurisdictions and disciplines to work together in response to natural disasters and emergencies, including acts of terrorism. Some of the highlights include a unified approach to incident management, standard command and management structures, and emphasis on preparedness, mutual aid, and resource management [14]. The entities required to be NIMS compliant are governments and organizations that receive federal grants. The implications for NIMS compliance are broad and affect governments, corporations, and nongovernmental organizations. IMERT members are all NIMS compliant and have insight into the importance of an incident command structure to any response situation. In addition to the required course work, IMERT members are provided with numerous educational and training programs, many in collaboration with other agencies. Some examples of these programs are cadaver workshops that demonstrate anatomic aspects of certain IMERT clinical skills, IMERT-sponsored and -developed domestic preparedness courses, the annual IMERT conference, advanced hazmat life support, equipment training sessions, incident command training courses, explosives and bomb response programs, simulation mannequin workshops, and basic trauma life support through the International Trauma Life Support Organization, Advance Cardiac Life Support, and National Disaster Life Support programs.

The National Disaster Life Support program is worthy of further discussion. National Disaster Life Support program is a collaborative effort among the American Medical Association, the Medical College of Georgia, the University of Georgia, and the University of Texas, with federal appropriations managed by the Centers for Disease Control and Prevention. In 2004, the National Disaster Life Support educational consortium offered a train-the-trainer program for providers in Illinois. IMERT was in the unique position to extend this offer to their member leadership. As a result of that effort, two IMERT leaders, one of them an oral surgeon, became course directors and have been able to provide the coursework for members and other professionals in Illinois. The program provides varying levels of knowledge and skills in all hazards topics and response for the health care and non–health care community (core disaster life support) to the basic and advanced medical professional. The advance disaster life support course offers an advanced practicum using medical simulation mannequins and technology that are at the forefront of medical training [15–17]. The simulations include scenarios with CBRNE-related events. The Disaster

Emergency Medicine Readiness Training Center in Chicago, Illinois is one of the training sites. The Center has instructors and program directors who are also IMERT members. The Disaster Emergency Medicine Readiness Training Center has particular relevance to the dental community. It is housed in the University of Illinois, College of Dentistry. The Disaster Emergency Medicine Readiness Training Center prepares health care professionals within the Sate of Illinois, FEMA Region V, and the nation. It also focuses on the role of the oral health care professional in bioterrorism and disaster response [18]. It began with initial Health Resources Services Administration funds allocated by IDPH and funds from the Centers for Disease Control and Prevention, which gives validation toward the important leadership role that oral health care professionals can contribute to emergency response.

Credentialing and indemnification are two important factors in the provision of reliable emergency response in a mass casualty event. These issues were particularly evident on September 11, 2001, when medical providers responded to the World Trade Center attack without readily available credentials, insight to their level of training in disasters, lack of knowledge of command structure, and lack of oversight [19]. This led Congress to authorize federal authorities to assist states and territories in developing emergency systems for the advance registration of volunteer health professionals (ESAR-VHP). Through advance registration, it is proposed that volunteers will be vetted, trained, and mobilized more effectively during emergencies [20–22]. The end result is a reliable and identifiable health care professional capable of integrating into the overall response to an event with oversight by the sponsoring organization. IMERT's inherent structure has set forth the components necessary for meeting a program such as ESAR-VHP.

Although ESAR-VHP addresses the professional integrity of a health care volunteer, it does not address the liability issues. The legal environment of volunteer health care professionals is complex and ambiguous at best. Some recommendations proposed include minimum legal standards, balanced liability protections, and compensations for harms to volunteers [20]. The Illinois legislature has enacted several laws called Public Acts that address some of the challenges in meeting the legal protection of such volunteers. IMERT is covered under Public Act 92-597 or the IEMA Act last amended in June 2002. The state, under the IEMA Act, extends workman's compensation and liability coverage and reimbursement for the response if there is a gubernatorial disaster declaration [23]. This has offered a certain level of comfort for IMERT volunteers, their employers, and their families. Another legislative support for emergency responders is Public Act 94-409 signed into law in August 2005, which includes the definition of a dental emergency responder, which modifies the scope of practice of dentists in Illinois who respond to emergencies from local to state. The dental emergency responder is a dentist or dental hygienist "acting within the bounds of his or her license when providing care during a declared local, state or national emergency" [12]. This law allows for legal recognition of a dental professional as a valuable health care resource in a disaster.

Illinois medical emergency response team relationships and partnerships

IMERT's success is the result of the diverse partnerships and collaborations formed with other agencies and organizations. These relationships have benefited IMERT by shared exercises and educational opportunities. They also provide a source of expertise in advancing different sectors and goals of IMERT administration. The dental profession's abilities to help facilitate some of these contacts have been a great asset. Some of these partnerships and their benefits to IMERT are discussed.

IMERT is part of the integrated disaster planning of Illinois. It is under the direction of IDPH and IEMA. IEMA is a lead agency in any disaster response and the state's emergency operations center. The state also has an entity entitled the Illinois Terrorism Task Force. As of 2005, the Illinois Terrorism Task Force had 54 agencies and associations that represent response disciplines from all parts of the state [24]. IDPH and IEMA are two of the partners. This task force permits multiple agencies and disciplines to share information and strategic planning for potential disaster and mass casualty-related events. The leadership and relationship of IDPH with the overall preparedness of the state have been well described [25]. Partnership with the IDPH-sponsored EMS for children has provided IMERT with much-needed pediatric expertise and as a potential opportunity for dentists.

Another organization that has been a valuable support for IMERT is the Illinois Fire Services Association and the Illinois Fire Chiefs Association. Many IMERT members are from urban and rural fire departments, including EMTs and paramedics. The support of the Illinois Fire Chiefs Association has permitted members to be active participants and have job protection should they be deployed. Illinois fire leadership also has partnered with IEMA through the Mutual Aid Box Alarm System, which is a mutual aid organization among most fire departments in Illinois with contractual agreements that provide assistance to other fire departments when their local resources are strained or overwhelmed. It is a unique program that began in the 1960s and has partnered with IEMA to become an important resource for the state, providing additional firefighter and EMS resources, including personnel and equipment, when needed. Surge requests can bring numerous firefighters and EMTs to the scene.

Another important partnership is with the Illinois College of Emergency Physicians, the state chapter of the American College of Emergency Physicians. IDPH contracted with Illinois College of Emergency Physicians in 2000 to provide administrative support for IMERT and develop the educational portions under the initial Centers for Disease Control and Prevention grant. This relationship continues into 2007. The Illinois College of

Emergency Physicians provides meetings rooms, administrative support, and accounting of grant funds that provide financial support for IMERT. It also has provided information technology support for the many of IMERT's activities, including IMERT's Web page. The Illinois College of Emergency Physicians collaborates with IDPH in other arenas (eg, the state's trauma advisory board, the EMS forum, and the EMS advisory council). The college is a positive fit for the mission of IMERT because many of the members are part of the emergency response system of the state.

Nurses also play a vital role in the development and leadership for IMERT and INVENT. The latter organization is nurse led with medical oversight and command via the IMERT command staff. INVENT was created through Health Resources Services Administration funds granted to the Illinois Emergency Nurse Association. INVENT has provided continuation of care and recovery missions after an initial deployment of IMERT. Their team members also provide educational and training support for many IMERT-related events.

There is mutual exchange of knowledge and expertise with the Illinois Poison Center, which is also an integral part of the overall emergency response of IDPH. The Illinois Poison Center has shared educational programs with IMERT, including content for bioterrorism, pandemic flu, radiologic terrorism, and provision of the advanced hazmat life support course for members. It is also a reliable, knowledgeable, and prompt information resource for IMERT medical members when seeking out information.

The University of Illinois, College of Dentistry has provided National Disaster Life Support programs and a resource for recruiting oral health care professions to volunteerism. IMERT also has established relationships with numerous educational organizations. Governor's State University and Southern Illinois University, Carbondale have provided their facilities and teaching staff in supporting the cadaver sessions. IMERT has delivered their domestic preparedness course to numerous medical schools, nursing programs, and EMT programs throughout the state. Emergency medicine residents from several training programs (eg, Stroger Hospital of Cook County, University of Illinois, Chicago, and Chicago College of Osteopathic Medicine) have been trained to be IMERT volunteers. Students from area public health programs have interned with IMERT. It is hoped that more dental students and professionals will be attracted to these relationships. These multiple partnerships and relationships keep the concept of IMERT vibrant.

Levels of activation

IMERT can be activated on several levels. Each event leads to after-action reports that become a lessons learned guide for the team and its command staff. These levels include drills/exercises, predeployments, and deployments. It is understood that actual deployments would not be frequent, because IMERT by definition is a resource when local resources become exhausted or overwhelmed. Local and regional (eg, county government) response is often adequate and maintains appropriate command of an event site [26]. Large-scale disasters are uncommon. Illinois has not had an earthquake since the late 1800s, and tornadoes, although devastating, are limited in occurrence. Other natural disasters with significant regional impact are also infrequent (eg, Midwest flood of 1993 and heat crisis of 1995). It is fortunate that these events are few, but to be fully ready to stand up for an event, preparedness response teams must train regularly. IMERT has actively sought integration with numerous exercises throughout the state with the support and approval of IDPH and IEMA. Drills and exercises are scheduled throughout the year. Some are large-scale in terms of personnel and equipment and various interagency activities. Some are "table-top" and test specific protocols of IMERT. An example of a table-top exercise would be a communication drill to test the dispatch system that partners with IMERT and the response readiness of team members on call in real-time. Predeployments are situations in which state authority has recognized a potential need for additional medical support (eg, an impending weather-related impact to a large region of the state). Deployments are actual declared disasters or events by the authority of the governor's office, and IMERT members are actually triggered to respond. Upon confirmed deployment, members are protected legally and medically by the state during the interval of response.

Predeployment exercises took place in 2005 in response to a terrorist event and a natural disaster. During the London train bombings, IMERT increased the number of teams on call to maintain a heightened alert for immediate activation. Each member was contacted and his or her ability to be deployed was verified. In preparation for Hurricane Rita, IMERT created a standby team of more than 100 members ready to be deployed to the Gulf region if requested by the governor's office. IMERT's mission is to be prepared for the state; on-call members are always to remain within its borders. In the rare circumstance that deployment occurs beyond state geographic boundaries, members not on call are requested to volunteer additional time only with release by their respective employers. Dental profession members have been supportive in all these efforts.

Although actual deployments are infrequent, IMERT readily lends itself to the needs of the state and has gained much in terms of experience and lessons learned to improve the organization. In April 2005, IMERT deployed for the Abraham Lincoln Presidential Library Museum opening in Springfield, Illinois. The celebration had a high potential for a terrorist threat as a result of the large contingent of governmental dignitaries, including current and former presidents and the large public attendance. This exercise allowed IMERT to work intimately with other agencies at the "ground" level (eg, Army Civil Support Team, state WMD, and local EMS) and up through IDPH at the emergency operations center.

IMERT was deployed out of state in 2004 in response to Hurricane Katrina. Illinois sent IMERT via a mutual aid contract between states called the Emergency Management Assistance Compact, which is a legislatively enacted agreement between states to share resources in times of disaster. In 1996, Congress ratified the Emergency Management Assistance Compact (Public Law 104–321), making it the first national disaster compact since the Civil Defense Compact of 1950 [27]. It began in the southeastern states in response to the regional impact of hurricanes. It would augment national support. Assets, including personnel and equipment caches deployed, are legally protected by the originating state. Reimbursement is extended upon receipt of federal disaster funds distributed to the requesting state [28–30]. Forty-nine states and several US territories have established Emergency Management Assistance Compact agreements.

When Hurricane Katrina devastated the Gulf region, one of the assets Louisiana requested was medical support. Illinois had been one of the few states with a trained, credentialed, and organized medical response team, IMERT. Under the direction of IDPH, IEMA, and the Illinois state emergency operations center, IMERT sent a total of 54 members to Louisiana State University in the state capital of Baton Rouge. The university's athletic facilities were designated as the receiving center for hurricane evacuees from New Orleans (eg, Superdome, convention center, airport, nursing homes, area hospitals, and residential homes). Immediately upon arrival, the first group of 11 members established command in collaboration with local incident command and unified command from the Louisiana emergency operations center. An additional 43 members were requested within hours of arrival when the need for additional IMERT support became evident. IMERT also partnered intimately with several agencies on site, especially the New Mexico DMAT, US Public Health Services personnel, FEMA, local EMS, local public health, Louisiana State University personnel, and area hospitals. IMERT and their partners initiated mass triage protocols, medical treatment, and disposition planning. At the end of the 1-week operation, approximately 15,000 persons were triaged. More than 6000 were treated and transported to appropriate medical facilities (ie, tertiary hospitals and long-term care facilities). Medical care ranged from medication refills to critical emergency care. This operation was well described by one of the IMERT nurse commanders [31]. The deployment was a watershed event for IMERT and led to accelerated growth in volunteers and equipment. Opportunities like these demonstrate the need for increased involvement of dental professionals and their expertise (Fig. 4).

An organization structured like IMERT can provide the vehicle for oral health care professionals to become part of a comprehensive and coordinated response. It also can provide the necessary training and experience to individuals who wish to provide volunteer services to their communities.

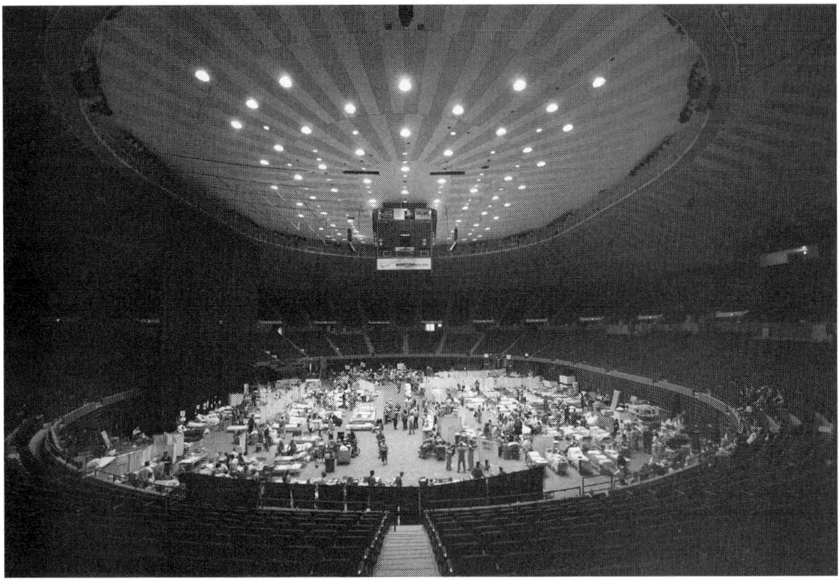

Fig. 4. Louisiana State University athletic center: IMERT operations for Hurricane Katrina in Baton Rouge, Louisiana (September 2005).

Ten IMERT dentists participated in various predeployments and deployments in 2006.

Future directions

IMERT has grown exponentially since its humble beginnings in 1999. Through sustained public health support and strong partnerships, it has become a reliable resource for Illinois. There are many areas to improve and discover as IMERT continues to mature. The organization is positioned to lend itself to rigorous research, including metric tools that can perform objective measures of the adequacy of protocols and response dynamics. It is hoped that sustained funding will be maintained. IMERT also can serve as a model for other states to develop similar programs and showcase oral health inclusion in a response. Health care professions have begun to realize that CBRNE and emergency response training are important curriculum additions, and it has been recognized in medical, dental, and nursing schools [32]. New York University College of Dentistry successfully introduced a senior course into its curriculum [33]; it is already an integral part of EMT training. Disasters of all causes have been part of civilization, so it behooves communities to continually improve their level of preparedness as more is learned about response, mitigation, and recovery. Introducing these concepts in early professional curriculum provides a potential pool of individuals well prepared in disaster management and leadership.

Another facet of team growth is the possible development of an Illinois DMAT. A DMAT team is another avenue of clinical participation for dentists in Illinois. Dentists also have been active in federal disaster mortuary operational response teams since its inception in the 1990s [32].

IMERT leadership has established numerous mutually beneficial partnerships, some of which could be expanded. The IMERT and disaster emergency medicine readiness training linkage with the College of Dentistry lends itself to fertile ground for educating and recruiting dental and oral hygienist students. Interstate partnership also will be explored to allow better knowledge of available resources in other states and opportunities to test the capabilities of Emergency Management Assistance Compact agreements. IMERT cannot exist solely within the realm of health care professionals and responders. The community at large also must be cognizant of the readiness and preparedness available to them at times of crisis. Planning with state, county, and local public health officials to inform and educate the public contributes to IMERT's success and acceptance when they respond to an event.

Summary

IMERT has grown from an initial team of approximately 200 volunteers to more than 1000 volunteers. As of 2006, there were 18 dental health professionals fully trained and credentialed; their participation has been invaluable. The current dental profession volunteers have served as role models for other members. Participation in drills, predeployments, and deployments can only add to the experience of IMERT members and give rise to its continuing quality improvement. IMERT members are encouraged to inform its leadership of potential exercises in their communities that may play a role in medical response. The future of IMERT is filled with opportunities and interjected with challenges. To provide a systematic approach, the IMERT executive council recently submitted to IDPH several goals it feels are worthy of accomplishing in a "5-year" plan. One of those goals is to increase the involvement of oral health care professionals through their educational institutions and organizations.

References

[1] DHHS. Disaster medical assistance teams (DMAT). Available at: http://www.oep-ndms.dhhs.gov/teams/dmat.html. Accessed July 13, 2007.

[2] Mann NC, MacKenzie E, Anderson C. Public health preparedness for mass-casualty events: a 2002 state-by-state assessment. Prehospital Disaster Med 2004;19(3):245–55.

[3] Tucker JB. National health and medical services response to incidents of chemical and biological terrorism. JAMA 1997;278(5):362–8.

[4] Illinois Medical Emergency Response Team. Available at: www.imert.org. Accessed July 13, 2007.

[5] Rhodes JD, Carafano JJ. State and regional responses to disasters: solving the 72-hour problem. The Heritage Foundation 2006. Available at: http://www.nyu.edu/ccpr/Survey_article_wp_final.pdf.
[6] Illinois State Weapons of Mass Destruction Team. Available at: http://www.ready.illinois.gov/ittf/2002reviews.htm. Accessed July 13, 2007.
[7] Illinois Urban Search and Rescue Team. Available at: http://www.il-tf-1.org. Accessed July 13, 2007.
[8] Illinois State Dental Society. Supply of practicing dentists in Illinois. Available at: http://www.isds.org/lawsLegislation/positstatements/SupplyDent.pdf. Accessed July 13, 2007.
[9] Psoter WJ, Glotzer D, Rekow D, et al. Enhancing medical and public health capabilities during times of crisis: a summary report on the expansion of the role of dentists and their enhancement of the medical surge response. New York: Department of Justice; 2003. p. 1–22.
[10] Janousek JT, Jackson DE, De Lorenzo RA, et al. Mass casualty triage knowledge of military medical personnel. Mil Med 1999;164(5):332–5.
[11] Psoter WJ, Alfano MC, Rekow ED. Meeting a disaster's medical surge demand: can dentists help? J Calif Dent Assoc 2004;32(8):694–700.
[12] Colvard MD, Lampiris LN, Cordell GA, et al. The dental emergency responder: expanding the scope of dental practice. J Am Dent Assoc 2006;137(4):468–73.
[13] Katz AR, Nekorchuk DM, Holck PS, et al. Dentists' preparedness for responding to bioterrorism: a survey of Hawaii dentists. J Am Dent Assoc 2006;137(4):461–7.
[14] Federal Emergency Management Agency. National incident management system. Available at: http://www.fema.gov/emergency/nims/index.shtm. Accessed February 3, 2007.
[15] Issenberg SB, McGaghie WC, Hart IR, et al. Simulation technology for health care professional skills training and assessment. JAMA 1999;282(9):861–6.
[16] Reznek M, Harter P, Krummel T. Virtual reality and simulation: training the future emergency physician. Acad Emerg Med 2002;9(1):78–87.
[17] Small SD, Wuerz RC, Simon R, et al. Demonstration of high-fidelity simulation team training for emergency medicine. Acad Emerg Med 1999;6(4):312–23.
[18] Disaster Emergency Medicine Readiness Training Center. Available at: http://dentistry.uic.edu/research/demrt/. Accessed July 13, 2007.
[19] Cone DC, Weir SD, Bogucki S. Convergent volunteerism. Ann Emerg Med 2003;41(4):457–62.
[20] Hodge JG Jr, Gable LA, Calves SH. Volunteer health professionals and emergencies: assessing and transforming the legal environment. Biosecur Bioterror 2005;3(3):216–23.
[21] Hoard ML, Tosatto RJ. Medical Reserve Corps: strengthening public health and improving preparedness. Disaster Manag Response 2005;3(2):48–52.
[22] Schultz CH, Stratton SJ. Improving hospital surge capacity: a new concept for emergency credentialing of volunteers. Ann Emerg Med 2006.
[23] State of Illinois. 2002 ITTF accomplishments. Available at: http://www.ready.illinois.gov/ittf/2002accomplishments.htm. Accessed July 13, 2007.
[24] State of Illinois Homeland Security. ITTF membership. Available at: http://www.ready.illinois.gov/ittf/membership.htm. Accessed July 13, 2007.
[25] Turnock BJ. Public health preparedness at a price: Illinois. New York: The Century Foundation; 2004. p. 1–39.
[26] Waugh WL. Regionalizing emergency management: countries as state and local government. Public Adm Rev 1994;(3):253–8.
[27] Illinois Terrorism Task Force Training Committee Report, December 2005. Available at: http://www.fsi.uiuc.edu/. Accessed July 13, 2007.
[28] Hodge JG Jr, O'Connell JP. The legal environment underlying influenza vaccine allocation and distribution strategies. J Public Health Manag Pract 2006;12(4):340–8.
[29] Waugh WL. The political costs of failure in the Katrina and Rita disasters. Ann Am Acad Pol Soc Sci 2006;604(1):10–25.

[30] Lowenberg TJ. The role of the national guard in national defense and homeland security. National Guard Association of the United States. September 2005;1–7.
[31] Connelly M. IMERT deployment to Baton Rouge, Louisiana in response to Hurricane Katrina, 2005. Disaster Manag Response 2006;4(1):4–11.
[32] Markenson D, DiMaggio C, Redlener I. Preparing health professions students for terrorism, disaster, and public health emergencies: core competencies. Acad Med 2005;80(6):517–26.
[33] Glotzer DL, More FG, Phelan J, et al. Introducing a senior course on catastrophe preparedness into the dental school curriculum. J Dent Educ 2006;70(3):225–30.

ELSEVIER
SAUNDERS

THE DENTAL CLINICS OF NORTH AMERICA

Dent Clin N Am 51 (2007) 895–898

Index

Note: Page numbers of article titles are in **boldface** type.

doi:10.1016/S0011-8532(07)00083-3

Moving?

Make sure your subscription moves with you!

To notify us of your new address, find your **Clinics Account Number** (located on your mailing label above your name), and contact customer service at:

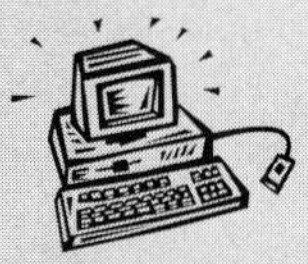

E-mail: elspcs@elsevier.com

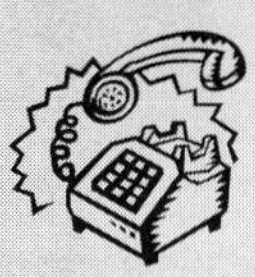

800-654-2452 (subscribers in the U.S. & Canada)
407-345-4000 (subscribers outside of the U.S. & Canada)

Fax number: 407-363-9661

Elsevier Periodicals Customer Service
6277 Sea Harbor Drive
Orlando, FL 32887-4800

*To ensure uninterrupted delivery of your subscription, please notify us at least 4 weeks in advance of move.

ELSEVIER

United States Postal Service

Statement of Ownership, Management, and Circulation (All Periodicals Publications Except Requestor Publications)

1. Publication Title Dental Clinics of North America	2. Publication Number 5 6 6 - 4 8 0	3. Filing Date 9/14/07
4. Issue Frequency Jan, Apr, Jul, Oct	5. Number of Issues Published Annually 4	6. Annual Subscription Price $171.00

7. Complete Mailing Address of Known Office of Publication (*Not printer*) (*Street, city, county, state, and ZIP+4*)

Elsevier Inc.
360 Park Avenue South
New York, NY 10010-1710

Contact Person
Stephen Bushing
Telephone (Include area code)
215-239-3688

8. Complete Mailing Address of Headquarters or General Business Office of Publisher (*Not printer*)

Elsevier Inc., 360 Park Avenue South, New York, NY 10010-1710

9. Full Names and Complete Mailing Addresses of Publisher, Editor, and Managing Editor (*Do not leave blank*)

Publisher (*Name and complete mailing address*)

John Schrefer , Elsevier, Inc., 1600 John F. Kennedy Blvd. Suite 1800, Philadelphia, PA 19103-2899

Editor (*Name and complete mailing address*)

John Vassallo, Elsevier, Inc., 1600 John F. Kennedy Blvd. Suite 1800, Philadelphia, PA 19103-2899

Managing Editor (*Name and complete mailing address*)

Catherine Bewick, Elsevier, Inc., 1600 John F. Kennedy Blvd. Suite 1800, Philadelphia, PA 19103-2899

10. Owner (*Do not leave blank. If the publication is owned by a corporation, give the name and address of the corporation immediately followed by the names and addresses of all stockholders owning or holding 1 percent or more of the total amount of stock. If not owned by a corporation, give the names and addresses of the individual owners. If owned by a partnership or other unincorporated firm, give its name and address as well as those of each individual owner. If the publication is published by a nonprofit organization, give its name and address.*)

Full Name	Complete Mailing Address
Wholly owned subsidiary of	4520 East-West Highway
Reed/Elsevier, US holdings	Bethesda, MD 20814

11. Known Bondholders, Mortgagees, and Other Security Holders Owning or Holding 1 Percent or More of Total Amount of Bonds, Mortgages, or Other Securities. If none, check box → None

Full Name	Complete Mailing Address
N/A	

12. Tax Status (*For completion by nonprofit organizations authorized to mail at nonprofit rates*) (*Check one*)
The purpose, function, and nonprofit status of this organization and the exempt status for federal income tax purposes:
Has Not Changed During Preceding 12 Months
Has Changed During Preceding 12 Months (*Publisher must submit explanation of change with this statement*)

PS Form **3526**, September 2006 (Page 1 of 3 (Instructions Page 3)) PSN 7530-01-000-9931 **PRIVACY NOTICE**: See our Privacy policy in www.usps.com

13. Publication Title
Dental Clinics of North America

14. Issue Date for Circulation Data Below
July 2007

15. Extent and Nature of Circulation			Average No. Copies Each Issue During Preceding 12 Months	No. Copies of Single Issue Published Nearest to Filing Date
a. Total Number of Copies (*Net press run*)			2400	2300
b. Paid Circulation (By Mail and Outside the Mail)	(1)	Mailed Outside-County Paid Subscriptions Stated on PS Form 3541. (*Include paid distribution above nominal rate, advertiser's proof copies, and exchange copies*)	1131	1100
	(2)	Mailed In-County Paid Subscriptions Stated on PS Form 3541 (*Include paid distribution above nominal rate, advertiser's proof copies, and exchange copies*)		
	(3)	Paid Distribution Outside the Mails Including Sales Through Dealers and Carriers, Street Vendors, Counter Sales, and Other Paid Distribution Outside USPS®	479	510
	(4)	Paid Distribution by Other Classes Mailed Through the USPS (e.g. First-Class Mail®)		
c. Total Paid Distribution (*Sum of 15b (1), (2), (3), and (4)*) →			1610	1610
d. Free or Nominal Rate Distribution (By Mail and Outside the Mail)	(1)	Free or Nominal Rate Outside-County Copies Included on PS Form 3541	84	64
	(2)	Free or Nominal Rate In-County Copies Included on PS Form 3541		
	(3)	Free or Nominal Rate Copies Mailed at Other Classes Mailed Through the USPS (e.g. First-Class Mail)		
	(4)	Free or Nominal Rate Distribution Outside the Mail (Carriers or other means)		
e. Total Free or Nominal Rate Distribution (Sum of 15d (1), (2), (3) and (4)			84	64
f. Total Distribution (Sum of 15c and 15e) →			1694	1674
g. Copies not Distributed (See instructions to publishers #4 (page #3)) →			706	626
h. Total (Sum of 15f and g)			2400	2300
i. Percent Paid (15c divided by 15f times 100) →			95.04%	96.18%

16. Publication of Statement of Ownership

If the publication is a general publication, publication of this statement is required. Will be printed in the **October 2007** issue of this publication.

Publication not required

17. Signature and Title of Editor, Publisher, Business Manager, or Owner

Jean Fanucci – Executive Director of Subscription Services

Date: September 14, 2007

I certify that all information furnished on this form is true and complete. I understand that anyone who furnishes false or misleading information on this form or who omits material or information requested on the form may be subject to criminal sanctions (including fines and imprisonment) and/or civil sanctions (including civil penalties).

PS Form **3526**, September 2006 (Page 2 of 3)